I0066657

The GIFT

Kochouseph Chittilappilly is an industrialist, a philanthropist, a humanist and a bestselling author. He is the founder of V-Guard Industries Ltd and the popular amusement parks, Wonderla and Veega Land Developers Pvt Ltd.

Kochouseph was born in Kerala into a traditional agricultural family. He holds a Master's degree in Physics and began his career as a supervisor in an electronics company. He is the recipient of many awards for his exemplary contributions in business and philanthropy. He is happily married with two sons and two grandchildren.

The
GIFT

How I Gave Away
A **Kidney** And Got
Richer At **Heart**

Kochouseph Chittilappilly

RUPA

This is a Print On Demand copy and hence does not have special finishing on the cover.

Published by
Rupa Publications India Pvt. Ltd 2016
7/16, Ansari Road, Daryaganj
New Delhi 110002

Sales centres:
Allahabad Bengaluru Chennai
Hyderabad Jaipur Kathmandu
Kolkata Mumbai

Copyright © Kochouseph Chittilappilly 2016

The views and opinions expressed in this book are the author's own and the facts
are as reported by him which have been verified to the extent possible, and the
publishers are not in any way liable for the same.

While every effort has been made to verify the authenticity of the information
contained in this book, the publisher and the author are in no way liable for the
use of the information contained in this book.

All rights reserved.
No part of this publication may be reproduced, transmitted,
or stored in a retrieval system, in any form or by any means, electronic, mechanical,
photocopying, recording or otherwise,
without the prior permission of the publisher.

ISBN: 978-81-291-3959-7

Second impression 2016

10 9 8 7 6 5 4 3 2

The moral right of the author has been asserted.

This book is sold subject to the condition that it shall not, by way of trade or
otherwise, be lent, resold, hired out, or otherwise circulated, without the publisher's
prior consent, in any form of binding or cover
other than that in which it is published.

Contents

Foreword

I met Kochouseph Chittilappilly (KC) at an event organized by the Kerala Management Association in Cochin where I was invited to speak on my latest book, *The Elephant Catchers*, that dwelt on the subject of building scale in enterprise. The disarmingly unassuming KC was introduced to me as 'the legendary but reclusive founder of V-Guard, who is also the humanitarian who has given a kidney away to someone he doesn't know!'

The word V-Guard instantly rang a bell.

In the India of pre-economic liberalization days of the 1990s, there were very few companies that were the bellwethers of quality. V-Guard was one such company. In a fiercely competitive, global economy, quality is imperative. It is a term dictated by the consumer. However in the protected economy of yore, if you knew how to manage the system, it was a mere option. With that backdrop, V-Guard became more than just a voltage stabilizer. Its products did not ever fail. Yet no one knew about the man behind it. Even as the company, first started in 1977 with a loan of ₹100,000 and just two other workers, has today become a publicly listed ₹1750 crore enterprise, very few know who KC is. In our world, success of his magnitude brings both narcissism and megalomania, not desire for personal obscurity and a desire to give everything away.

When I had met KC, I somewhat knew about the philanthropic work he did but I was not aware that he had donated a kidney to a stranger. At the event, we shook hands and I told him how impressed I was with V-Guard as a fellow entrepreneur and a business writer. However I did make references about the kidney he had donated. I needed time to absorb the information, I did not want to be superficial about it. After the event, we went our own ways.

Several days later, I received a mail from him. He asked me if I would read a manuscript on his story about why and how he gave a kidney away. In the normal course of things, I decline requests for reading manuscripts because I cannot do justice to them, given my own commitments at work and the pressure of my own writing. However given the backdrop of the meeting, my admiration for his enterprise and the very unusual subject at hand, I said I would. When the soft copy of the book arrived, I read the first page and just could not keep it down. I was spellbound with many things; the story itself and more importantly, the very subject of cadaver donation about which both society and the medical community remains in vast ignorance.

For a country of 1.3 billion and more, it is not an esoteric subject. It could mean the difference between life and death for someone you know personally. After reading the book, the first thought that came to my mind was that it must spread far and wide, that it must be read by people from all walks of life about a little known subject of this magnitude. I asked KC to get a professional editor for the book and look for a good publisher in whose hands the message of the book would go far and wide. I am delighted that it is happening today.

The Gift is a book on humanity. It is a book that restores faith in the power of good at a time when indiscriminate greed and violence, both in thought and deed, has overtaken people and few have the time to pause and reflect. *The Gift* is also a book on what business leadership should be all about in a country like India. Business leaders are social leaders as well. They must see the purpose of business and the power of wealth as turners of the wheel of wellbeing for all people. KC is a shining example of that.

I am delighted that *The Gift* is in your hands right at this moment, and I hope you will treasure its message in your heart, that you would emulate KC's example in your own way, and make an impact on people you do not know and may never meet in your life!

Subroto Bagchi
28 June 2015

Chapter 1

The Beginning

I remember the big white lights. I remember eight or nine men and women standing around me dressed in green cloaks. Their faces were covered with surgical masks. I could only see their eyes peering down at me. Then it all started to get blurry. While slipping away, I began to wonder why I was there.

What had brought me to that surgical table under those bright lights?

It had all started with a thought that had floated into my mind about eight months ago. One tiny thought. In the intervening months, it had grown and now I lay naked under a green cloak, surrounded by strangers wearing masks and uniforms. I began slipping, drifting to a white phantom land under the blinding light. I wondered how big the knife was going to be. I thought of my beloved wife Sheela.

I mumbled to myself, 'Be calm, be calm, everything's going to be fine.'

In life, we do not know how it will all end. We can only hope for the best. The adventure that brought me to this surgery table, started off as a casual conversation in June 2010. Before I recount that conversation, let me tell you a little bit about myself and my family.

I was born in a sleepy village called Parappur situated about sixteen kilometres away from Thrissur, a temple town in Kerala. To many of those in Mumbai and New Delhi, Kerala itself is a sleepy place. Consider then a small village tucked far away from the hustle and bustle of the big towns in Kerala. In my mind, I can still see the green fields. At dawn, we walked barefoot on the soft green meadows through the misty whiteness, happy and contented. Fields of paddy stretched all around us. Our days began with the sounds of the quacking of ducks and the crowing of roosters. Tamarinds and mangoes and tender green banana plantains grew everywhere.

Ours was a traditional Christian farmer's family. My family relied on our bullock cart for our family trips. Our home did not have electricity and when going out in the late evenings, a lit slender bundle of dried coconut plantain leaves served as a torch. At home, we used kerosene lamps. We never wore slippers. Even if we owned a pair, it would lie unused at home while our feet grew bigger with each passing day.

Our father believed in us being an integral part of the

village community. If, for some reason, our friends in the neighbourhood could not go for a school picnic, he would tell us to stay back too. Austerity and care for others were the beliefs that we grew up with all the way up to our adulthood and even later. This simplicity has stayed with me even today, when I sit atop a ₹1750 crore enterprise. I trust my simple ways. It was natural that I grew up into a caring and careful man.

In 1977, I set up V-Guard Industries as a small manufacturing unit with money borrowed from my father. I had just two unskilled workers. Since then my company has grown remarkably. It has received praise from shores beyond our own for the progress it has made. From ₹300 crores in 2008–09, revenues have grown to ₹1750 crores in 2014–15. We were already riding on an impressive wave of success in manufacturing and selling India's most respected household brand of stabilizers and electrical goods when we opened the country's leading amusement park, Veegaland (which has been renamed as Wonderla). Over the years many awards have come my way like the Manorama Newsmaker of the Year, Business Man of the Millennium, Tourism Man of the Year, Top Income Tax Payer, amongst many others. I am grateful for these honours and the moments.

If you ask me, I am a first-generation businessman who turned simple ideas into India's future-ready businesses. For me, life is about possibilities.

Coming back to the story of how I ended up on the

surgical table, I have to take you back thirteen years, to the day my elder son Arun came home and said he was in love with a girl named Priya. He said he wanted to marry her.

Priya was her parent's only child. From what Arun told us, she sounded like the perfect match in every way except for one reason. Her mother Valsa had a failing kidney. My first response was to tell Arun to reconsider his decision.

I am a careful man. I believe I have made some wise moves in life. I have also committed a few mistakes. Such trials and errors make a man more careful. Our flagship company, V-Guard, was flourishing. My entrepreneurial status across the nation was quite gratifying. I had plans for my sons in my company, if they were willing. My second son Mithun was then studying in the final year of college towards a B.Com degree. I only wanted the best for my sons. Arun's choice to marry this girl could have been perfect tidings for us all or at least desirable on its own terms. However, like I said, when you are at the beginning, you don't know how it is all going to end. The girl he chose and the family he wanted to have the alliance with were truly noble. Yet I was not sure at that moment. I cautioned him. Arun stood there like a rock. Finally I realized that he was truly in love. My son had found his mate for life. It is a momentous time for us as parents to see their children choose their life partners.

A few weeks later, we called on Priya's parents. Her father, Captain Joseph (affectionately called Jocha at home), had been on a merchant navy ship once. He had since then become the CEO of a shipping company and was posted in Hong Kong. Jocha was a pleasant man, one who had seen the world; a jovial father who would treat you with his best wine stock. We also met Valsa. She was around forty-nine years old. She looked weak and quite ill. Till that day I had not known anyone in my close circle with a troubled kidney. I did not know how torturous the ailment could be for the person who was suffering from such a sickness. Till that time I had never had the time to even think of ailments.

Is it not common amongst us?

We go on living without giving much thought to our own vital organs. We all take our bodies for granted till something goes wrong. What does not worry us, is never remembered. Obviously, the kidney remained an old high school biology lesson for me, a name of an organ that I knew.

At Priya's home, we exchanged pleasantries with Jocha and Valsa. They treated us with a lot of affection. They were glad about the alliance. Priya was a charming woman. She was gentle and extremely well-mannered; born and bred in London. In them, I found an affectionate family. However I had not overcome my worries. I worried that Valsa's poor health would pile up on Priya's daily responsibilities.

Would it not be such an emotional challenge and in turn affect Arun and his life with Priya?

Any father in my shoes would have thought the same. Other than this bit, I was completely happy. I am a simple man and like to be in harmony with the world and my circumstances. I am also a father. I only wished for the wellbeing of my dear ones—be it my sons or my daughters-in-law or grandchildren.

The alliance now had the blessings of both families and Priya's parents began to visit us often. It was then that I began to see how much a kidney patient suffers. Valsa needed help to even get up from a chair. She could not climb up or down the stairs without two people holding her on either side. Her body had some swelling, easily visible, and she often looked pale. As the ailment worsened, they decided to do a kidney transplant. I was told that they had managed to find a donor. I kept wondering if Valsa would be healthy again. At times my doubt got replaced by worries.

Once the transplant surgery took place, Valsa's health transformed in a matter of days. Our families began going for trips together. On these trips, her cheerful demeanour was palpable and even infectious. For her, it was like a second life. Her pain gone, she was now literally on her feet. We were quite jubilant about her recovery. It was not just a passing euphoria. It gave birth to a renewed faith within me in medical science.

How could a surgery resurrect someone like this?

I became conscious about the power of medicines; about how health centres enlivened us. Babies are born every day in hospitals. All around the world, the bruised and the broken and the melancholic are resurrected by doctors and nurses.

Yet we also carry a sense of fear about those solemn white beds?

We still grow cold when a telephone call beckons us to a hospital. That is because hospitals are also a place for possible failures. They can bring us terrible news. News of impossibilities. News of bereavement.

Soon, the day of the wedding came. To our surprise, we found Valsa managing all the arrangements on her own. Jocha, as the head of the shipping company, was out of the country most of the time. Through her simple and earnest efforts, Valsa charmed and cheered us. After the wedding, we went on holidays with Valsa, Arun and Priya. All this while, I was also silently observing Valsa.

Following our vacation, Jocha and Valsa went on a trip to Alaska in the US. The lady who once fumbled to rise from a chair on her own, was doing adventure sports like white water rafting and hot air balloon rides. Months later, on our way to China we again touched down at Singapore to visit Valsa and Jocha as he had got transferred from Hong Kong to Singapore. Jocha was busy with his duties, but Valsa drove us around through the busy town. At home she cooked exotic dishes for us and entertained us with her wonderful sense of humour. She, at each turn, simply surprised us. I kept watching her and marvelled time and again on the capabilities of medical science. Normally, I wouldn't bet a penny on so-called miracles. This, I felt, was close to being one.

When Aarav was born to Priya and Arun, Valsa took over her duties like a wise and orderly grandmother. When Aarav was just four months old, he was diagnosed with a rare anomaly in his heart. It crushed us all. However strong a man I thought I was, I could not sleep properly worrying about my little grandson. His tiny heart had a hole. The doctors said he needed a surgery. It was a blow to us. My faith in healthcare was real but new to me. A challenge such as this, for my young grandson fighting for his life, was much larger than any faith I fancied I had in doctors. I would have traded this threat on Aarav with anything. Then again, Valsa stayed back in Bengaluru and was at Priya's side the whole time. Jocha was in Shanghai. Valsa was in hospital, day and night, assisting in every way possible. Aarav finally underwent an open heart surgery. I could barely sit or stand that whole day. Even when most of us were anxious, Valsa remained strong and calm. Aarav was put in the ICU for seven days straight. Our little Aarav eventually came through it like a charming angel. He recovered quickly. With tears of joy we held him close, thanking the medical fraternity once again for this marvellous feat.

Many years ago, I was a man of fear. I had fainted when I saw blood gushing out of a large cut on my brother's head. Decades later, after little Aarav and Valsa's recovery, my fears simply vanished. I was no longer averse to hospitals.

Chapter 2

Tides Turn

The good times, however, did not last long.

Within four months of Aarav's surgery, we got word from Hong Kong; Valsa had fallen ill again. Eight years had passed since Valsa's kidney transplant surgery. Then one day, Valsa just got sick. I was too naïve to understand such complications at that point. The details I learned about ailing kidneys and transplants came much later when I put myself under the bright lights of the operation theatre. Back then, I did not know much about it.

I learned from physicians and experts later that when a kidney gets transplanted, it works well for twelve to fifteen to twenty years in the recipient, and in some cases even longer. However if serious infections strike the person, the borrowed kidney will be the first organ to get affected. The body recognizes the transplanted organ as a foreign body that has come from outside and any viral attack on the body prompts it to dispel this foreign object first. It worked the same way in Valsa as well. One and a half years ago, she had got infected with pneumonia. Slowly, her kidney stopped functioning. Doctors suggested a second transplant. That was again news to me. We were told that there were patients who had undergone two or three transplants. The possibility of a second transplant gave us hope. Doctors ruled out the idea of Priya donating one of her kidneys to her mother. Their tissues and blood group didn't match. Jocha, being a heart patient, could not donate either. We had to start looking for fresh donors.

With the help of my brother in Thrissur we arranged a donor. We then began running around for the required permission and papers. Meanwhile the doctors ran fresh tests on Valsa. Repeated hospital routines vexed everyone. Priya kept coming down to Kochi from Bengaluru. We desperately wished to see a cheerful Valsa once again.

This was the time when I took one of the biggest decisions in my life. It was a decision that affected many lives around me. One day we were sitting in our living room talking about Priya's mother's condition.

I suddenly said, 'Maybe I should offer my kidney to somebody.'

There was stunned silence. At the time perhaps none of us, even I, did not realize the repercussions this thought would have. Priya was the only one who expressed her surprise. The others remained silent. I was just giving voice to a thought. Even now I don't know from where that strange idea came to me. Those who knew me understood that I'm not a man of whims and fancies. I'm a silent man following my own rules. I don't blurt out statements like that. It wasn't just about the family, it also had repercussions for our company.

V-Guard had ambitions to grow at the rate of 50 per cent annually with a planned scale to become a ₹5,000 crore enterprise. As long as I sat on top of such a commitment, answerable to hundreds of key stakeholders, thousands of shareholders, dealers and distributors across India, not to mention over a thousand employees, could I afford to entertain such thoughts?

Sometimes we speak the very moment we think of something. We spill out our half-formed thoughts. I don't normally do that. I let fully formed ideas sink in me and let them out after days of their formation. However, by then, I had seen both an ailing Valsa and a resurrected Valsa. I had seen what diseases could do to those who we love and hold close. This feeling of losing hope was worrying me. On the other hand, I was also seeking an answer on my part, about what I could do about such things.

Once I had articulated the thought for the first time, I pushed it a little further and said aloud that maybe I'll donate the kidney if someone pays some money to my father's trust. The C.T. Thomas Trust, in my father's name, was running a home for the destitute in my village. The home had around thirty-six inmates. The trust also adopted children in various parts of Kerala to educate them. It served people under the Below Poverty Line scheme to get life insurance, medical assistance and other support. It must have sounded like a weak joke for I heard a resounding silence. Then I pushed for the third time.

'If I am healthy, why not donate a kidney?'

Sheela sat looking as if she didn't even want to entertain such a thought. Priya chided me, saying they would not accept it from a sixty-year-old man.

I went on, 'Well, I'm only fifty-nine, let's ask the doctor.'

This time, Sheela and Arun answered me with their stares. They then went on about with their day. I guess Priya sat there feeling some empathy for that idea of mine. Neither of us said anything though. We let it go at that.

I've read somewhere that a little thought—or maybe one or two—can sometimes end up changing our entire lives. One thought could make us or break us. It could raise us or raze us down. That's the power of our thoughts. Some say thoughts become tangible; they earn a power on their own to grow within us. Decisions come from ideas. Actions follow. Men go to the moon following a thought, or launch a stabilizer business or open a water theme park following a thought.

Some also give away their organs following a thought.

At the time, I was writing my biography. It gave me a chance to introspect about my life. It set me thinking about my past, the paths I had taken, the things I had done, the life I had made around me. It helped me look at myself from the outside, like one would look at another person. I felt contented with my life.

V-Guard had moved beyond manufacturing just stabilizers and was manufacturing wires, cables and pump verticals. We had a good presence across India. We had a strong staff power of 1, 900 employees, a distribution network of 600 exclusive distributors, more than 192 service centres, 5, 500 channel partners, 29 branches and more than 20,000 retailers.

In 2007, we had listed V-Guards Industries on the Bombay Stock Exchange (BSE) and the IPO received a three out of five rating from Crisil. Our initial offer was oversubscribed by investors from Kerala. V-Guard was also listed on the National Stock Exchange of India Limited (NSE) at a premium of over 9.75 per cent against the issue price. These are business facts studded with technical terms. However the gist of it is that our business had grown satisfactorily, to say the least.

Naturally, I wondered if now was the time to do something more, something larger with my life. At that thought, I felt a slow stream of joy filling me. As days went by, I indulged myself with the idea of donating my kidney. The idea was growing stronger and I began to feel it was a wonderful proposition—to donate a vital organ for someone's good. I did not want any meanings layered to it. I wasn't being merciful to anyone. The last thing I had on my mind was the grand idea of benevolence. It was a thought as a healthy human being to do something for another human. If the doctors said one of my kidneys was good enough to be given away, well, it could be given away. Just like that.

Back then, my thought hadn't taken root in logic. It did not have the firmness into which it grew later. When I analyze it now, I think there was every chance I could have abandoned the idea in the very beginning. Not too many kidneys are donated in the country. In those days I used to interact with many doctors to check on Valsa's state of health and her progress. They were waiting for Valsa's health to improve so she could undergo a second surgery. The patient had to get healthier to withstand the operation. However to regain health, she needed her kidney. To put a kidney in her, she required better health. It was a catch-22 situation.

Then one day, Valsa died.

The news left us bereft. She died without getting a functional kidney. She had been promised a second transplant—a promise of a third life of sorts. However she had lost and regained and then lost again Priya crumbled. Valsa had died of cerebral haemorrhage. The transplant was scheduled for January 2010, but she passed away on 1 December 2009. Just about thirty days had separated her life from death.

I was upset because one fact stood there staring at me: Valsa would not have died if there was no delay in getting official approvals for the transplant. We had a willing legal donor. We had a patient gasping for life. Yet the government papers just didn't move in time. To get a right donor had taken time and by that time, her health had deteriorated. When we finally found a donor, doctors asked us to wait for another two months. Additionally, the sanctions had to come.

The thought that troubled me the most was that Valsa had died due to the non-availability of an organ, which I had the power to donate.

Why wouldn't any of these people, including me, who behave great and noble, consider donation?

This thought had begun to irritate me. It was not an easy thought. It was about knowing that you hold within yourself a certain power and yet not using it for someone's good. It is a thought that ought to unsettle every healthy, proactive male or female. We believe we have some responsibility to this world. Valsa's death was a nudge in that direction. I could see the possibility of several patients like Valsa dying. It would be like a man or a woman dying in public when all of us stood around and watched. It was akin to murder.

If it is in your capacity, in your power, then you have every right and duty to act.

Isn't that the essence of being human? Isn't that what makes us different from the beasts?

This compulsion for action, this feeling of needing to do something for the other, is what refines us, our personalities.

When Valsa died, I came to know more about the complications associated with kidney failure. It surprised me that she did not die from the failure of her kidney. Doctors told me that several kidney patients die because of cerebral haemorrhage. Continuous medications make a patient's blood vessels go thinner leading to sudden death.

We went through Valsa's funeral and the ceremonies with her memory fresh in our minds. Once it was all over, we got back to our normal lives. I began my hectic schedules with corporate meetings, board decisions, policy discussions and more. I had many responsibilities at the company. We were often in the limelight for the right reasons. All eyes of the media, business analysts and country's top investor advisors were constantly on us. My team was growing stronger. My heart was completely immersed in taking V-Guard further up. Yet, strangely, in the middle of all this, my wish to donate a kidney was growing its roots within me and had begun to fill my thoughts through days and nights.

Once again after a few weeks when I was with Sheela, I asked her, 'What if I donate a kidney when I am sixty and perfectly healthy?'

Sheela gave me that look again. That alerted me that I was to tread with care with such thoughts while at home. I smiled and changed the topic. Days went by. In our family meets, when my brothers and sisters were present, I would express my idea about donating a kidney aloud. It was like a child dropping a pebble in the pond. Then I'd cunningly keep quiet and listen to all the responses. If they were cold, I would ask them again.

'Well, why not?'

Some would laugh it off. Some would frown. I would withdraw after testing the waters. In truth, there was no compulsion anymore to keep this thought. Valsa's need for a kidney was over. It was not expected of a busy, successful entrepreneur to be holding such a wish in a serious way. The world around me naturally expected me to lead a 'normal' life enjoying my riches.

One day, while looking through some business papers in my office, I suddenly felt I should know if I'm healthy enough to donate a kidney. Whether my body would permit it. I did not want the thought to grow too large in me before I verified its viability. I'm a practical man. I did not want to lose sleep over some pipe dream with no end result.

Soon after, I met a doctor, a senior nephrologist in Thrissur. He was an elderly person and knew our family and Valsa's complete medical history. That was the first time I expressed this thought to someone outside my family. I shook hands with him and asked whether they would accept the kidney of a sixty-year-old. I was then fifty-nine. The good old doctor dismissed me with a smirk. 'No way!'

He said donors above fifty years of age are not encouraged since their health would not permit it.

It was like a sledgehammer falling on all my hopes. I was utterly disappointed.

Was my wholehearted wish going to remain a childish pretence?

I nodded and tried to change the topic with a smile. We

slipped into pleasantries. However, my despair began to burn me from inside. I hadn't failed like this before; failed before I had even properly started. Those who I had provoked with my question might now throw it back at me with a giggle.

'Oh, by the way, aren't you going to donate your kidney or something, Kochouseph?'

It was a hurtful thought. My wish may not have earned anyone's blessing, but somehow, somewhere I had fallen in love with it.

Chapter 3

How Life Arranges Us

We all come with varying capacities, be it physically and mentally. Yet we try to draw the best out of ourselves so we can be at par with everyone. For some, their body organs might be weak or non-functional. For others, disorders of body functions might trouble them. For some like me, there could be a learning disability of a minor degree.

When it came to numbers, for instance, if someone said sixty-nine, I would note it down as ninety-six. It might surprise many but it is true. For me, being a businessman always dealing with numbers, it could have been dangerous; or even comical. However it wasn't severe. I could manage it. As soon as it was diagnosed that I had dyslexia, I began to find ways to avoid big blunders. At times, I made the people around me repeat the numbers so that I could slowly engrave them in my head. I had the same problem when writing in English. I might write down 'leader' in place of 'dealer'. When I read documents I had written down, it would be nothing short of a carnival of errors. Sometimes my writing produced funny results; sometimes, the results were terrible. Most of the time, what I had taken down would be mismatched words or jumbled expressions. Even now my handwriting is illegible. Whatever writing I did would be marked and slashed, making it hard even for me to make out later.

This problem made me remain alert about my writing and also about what I spoke. I first go through what I wanted to say in my mind and then say it out loud. I read whatever I have written several times. Thus, my systemic error indirectly forced me to become cautious with my words and actions. I felt it was a blessing in disguise. Dyslexia, the disorder responsible for all this, helped me to become a stern reviewer of my own actions.

It took me many years to know that this was a disorder known to science. In fact, it was when my children began their schooling, that I learned the name of the disability. I could overcome it with my own methods.

However, what if I have within me a serious or more profound error in my faculties?

Such systemic errors could only be overcome with external support and medical assistance—like that of a kidney, for instance.

The medical advice I got from my good old friend hadn't

exactly cancelled away my desire entirely. What I heard from him about the age bar was a setback indeed. However, some part of me kept whispering that there could be another way, some way, some answer for me. These questions were constantly there at the back of my mind.

Normally, if I get hooked by an idea, I'll keep pursuing it. If something strikes me as worth pursuing, I have a habit of pushing it through. This was how I ran my company. We overcame several big challenges, including labour strikes and total shut down. Once I got down and unloaded the company material from the truck on my head, when the daily workers demanded an unreasonable amount of money. Even before all that, in the 1980s, trade union leaders threatened me. They warned they would kidnap my school-going sons if I didn't relent to their demands. The workers' strike of the 1980s forced me to shut down my units. However my spirit was strong. I had to come around in another way. That's when I thought of outsourcing the manufacturing to small enterprises, unaffected by labour issues. We trained women across Kerala to assemble stabilizers in their units. Now, there are some nineteen self-help groups in Kerala and thirty-five more spread across other southern states. Around 70 per cent of our turnover comes from outsourcing. The business world was not familiar with the concept of 'outsourcing' back then, when I implemented it. V-Guard can claim to be one of the pioneers.

Sometimes things take longer than expected to yield the

desired result. Many of my achievements happened because I refused to give up. Suppose you have set your mind on a venture and you want to win—but what you find is a shut door in front of you. My experience is that if you persist, two others will open. You wouldn't know how and where and when but the doors will open for sure. I like this philosophy. So even on the matter of donating my kidney, I was waiting to be fully convinced that I wasn't good enough to donate. I wanted to make sure before I ruled out the idea completely. I needed some clarity. At the same time, I did not want too many people to know that I had this wish. Or else a couple of phone calls would have settled the matter. However I feared the word might spread.

What if I wasn't physically fit to donate? Why set off crackers unnecessarily?

A few years ago, I had read in Paulo Coelho's book *The Alchemist* that the universe conspires and helps to make our intense desires come true. I cannot entirely claim to verify this belief with my experience. However I can happily say that there had been such interventions of what we call 'chance' or 'coincidences', that brought me closer to my goals. I'm sure most of us have had similar experience. In keeping with this belief, nothing better could have happened to me than the appearance of a concurring advisor.

Voila!

I have been a member of the Rotary Club since 1980. I was its president once but after my term, I became a regular member happily supporting its activities. Quite often, the club would invite specialists in various subjects to speak to us. The themes would vary. It would be mostly something that caught our attention or something quite topical. Sometimes, we accepted requests from professional organizations to send their orators to present their points of view. One day, a man named Shenoy walked into our club for such a lecture. He happened to be a campaigner for organ donations! Imagine my surprise. Here I was hoping against hope that my age would not hinder my wish to donate my organ and the perfect man had appeared to dispel the confusion clouding my mind!

Shenoy gave a terrific speech. He pulled apart our common superstitions about organs and organ donation and transplants. He was championing the idea of organ donation after death. His ideas simply seized me. I moved away from the usual chatter, picked a chair close to him and listened with rapt attention. I was hoping this man would mention something that would clear my doubts.

Is my wish to donate a kidney a legitimate idea? Did men of my kind and age have similar thoughts? Are there willing donors of kidneys in the country? Will I be barred from donating due to my age? Is this going to be too risky for me? Will I die?

There were too many queries and I was hoping that this evening I would finally have some proper answers.

Shenoy described why it was normal to donate one's organs. It was not a sacrifice, he said, because a donor is not losing anything. One could donate certain organs even while living. Or one could choose to donate upon one's death. This was in the case of organs like eyes. He said one could write a will to ensure that donation takes place. He also said there were organizations to help retrieve organs upon physical death or brain death. I was hearing just the things that I wanted to. I kept listening intently. Here was somebody who knew medico-legal ethics and the biological consequences of organ donation and was still recommending what I had begun to silently wish at heart. It was from that speech I came to know that even if we happened to be in coma or in case of our brain death, we could very well donate our liver, pancreas and even kidney. However, for practical purposes we ought to write a consent letter while we are alive. It made complete sense to me. As he pointed out, most often upon our death it would be our relatives and family who would decide on our behalf. So a written document is essential to record our wishes on the matter. If I remember right, he also recommended an organization named the Society for Organ Retrieval and Transplantation (SORT) for the same. He said that in certain countries, after one's death, the body became the property of the government and the government had all rights to retrieve the organs. He said in countries like France, Poland and Belgium, everyone is by default an organ donor, although some nations like Singapore allow opting out of it. If one met with an accident and is found dead, without any delay a team of well-equipped physicians arrive at the scene in a mobile unit and retrieve the organs before the person is functionally dead. He said it is mandatory there. Such an act can save many other lives. In New Zealand, when somebody applies for his driver's licence, the authorities check if he is willing to donate in case of such irreversible body conditions. All this was news to me—wonderful, heartening news. This man, Shenoy, was now rolling out a red carpet for making my wish come true.

It was like I was in Alice's wonderland and had gone down the rabbit hole. I forgot the surroundings—the club and the members sitting around me. I was totally engrossed in the most important talk I'd ever heard in that club. Till that day, I wasn't even aware of the phenomenon called 'brain death'. By definition, it means the brain and its stem irreversibly lose all their capacities to function. Legally, it is considered as death itself. However if the heart beats, with the aid of mechanical ventilation, some vital organs can be kept alive. Most organ retrieval happens at this stage. In such cases, even if the brain is dead, the heart and lungs could go on functioning and blood continues circulating within the body.

After all the biological details, Shenoy got down to practical matters. He said an application form should be filled by the one who wished to donate and entrust the form to family members. He even urged us to laminate the certificate and hang it on the wall. This would make it clear to people how much we want to donate. It also worked as some kind of emotional warranty among relatives to respect our wish and ensure the retrieval of organs in case of brain death. It is true that reminding anyone of the idea of death is an unpleasant business. However I agreed with Shenoy that this was a matter of practicality. It was part of planning for the future by a committed donor.

In a country like India, common religious beliefs and to a large extent, some superstitions prevent people from allowing such retrieval. It is totally unfortunate. The faithful should rethink.

Aren't even these religious rules originally meant for the wellbeing of the believers? Should such precepts become regressive forces that work against genuine human wishes?

When a brain dead person is cremated without taking out his kidney, such a precious and priceless organ is simply wasted away.

Does God wants us to be cremated with all our organs intact without a care if a fellow human being died due to lack of the organs we refused to donate?

Our willingness to see the dignity in donating an organ can save another life. Catholics believe in honouring the dignity of human life. Hinduism praises the sublimity involved in human birth when compared to the birth of a beast. Islam respects mankind.

So what comes between our choice to honour another life and our baseless fear?

It is only our ignorance; our unwillingness to reflect on our power to save a human. Just that. Lack of awareness can be as deadly as any disease. The churches and temples and mosques of this land can spread the message on organ donation loud and clear. One word from these opinion leaders would help spread the awareness like wildfire.

Some of us believe in life after death. However, some quite erroneously think that if they donate eyes, they will be reborn as blind.

What kind of logic is there in this?

Such superstitions go against even the Buddhist belief in rebirth. It is said that the Buddha himself wanted to put an end to the cycle of death and rebirth. He had mentioned that he himself had lived several thousand lives before this life as Siddhartha. These are mentioned in several books. I learned all this from those who know better. For example, Buddhists in Sri Lanka, following the word of their masters, staunchly believe in reincarnation and rebirth. Hence, it is common among the Sri Lankan Buddhists to donate their eyes. Not just monks, but even layman believers or followers of the path of the Buddha gladly donate their eyes after death. They believe that by donating their organs they are investing in the cosmic bank of goodness. Since it has become a mandatory religious rite, India gets a lot of donated eyes from Sri Lanka. In such a vast country like India that claims to be spiritual, we don't get enough eye donations! Let alone enough, we don't get even a fraction of the required number. Donation of eyes, liver, pancreas, kidney, etc., bring life, cheer, love and wonder into human lives.

We most often do nothing for the common good. We try to be practical and do things based on our own narrow-minded calculations. We hope to get more and to give less. Hence, voluntary donations are done only by a few. Though I'm against the state interfering in personal affairs, there are times when I wonder whether the federal government shouldn't consider a law by which organ donation is made mandatory.

Shenoy then told us that if one undergoes brain death, both the kidneys can be taken. This could give life to two people in place of one. He said kidneys could be donated even when one was alive and healthy. As I listened to his speech, my mind received more and more light and clarity on the subject. One and half months ago, I'd got confused by the casual advice of the doctor I had met. Now, my mind was clear. I could feel the happy ripples of my contentment. I was growing contented that my idea had the approval of this informed man. I remember asking him if there was any age restriction on the donor. He said he wasn't a physician but a social worker, yet he could ascertain that one can donate till sixty-five or seventy years of age. I had to hold back the joy that erupted within me. I couldn't show it as there were friends around.

How could I show my glee and escape without explaining my intentions?

I could hardly wait till I knew more.

When the meeting was over, some members were amused to see me checking this matter of age once again with Shenoy.

There were a few doctors among our members. Soon we moved out of the lecture room for our informal fellowship with those customary whisky glasses, sipping and breaking into group chuckles. These buddies of mine at the Rotary Club were good friends—decent people who are nice to each other in an urbane way. Most of us met for an hour every week. We shared a peg or two; then some private exchanges and some news and opinions. Some of our friendships go a long way back.

Then I sensed that they had a vague concern about my interest. A couple of doctor friends among them raised the topic.

'You were asking about the age bar. Are you up to some mischief?'

When they noticed that I wasn't entirely rebutting their statements, a kind of alarm crept on some faces. No! Seriously? Come on! I didn't want to start a wave of gossip. I smiled and even mumbled some excuses.

I think I got away.

I was good at changing topics by throwing around many anecdotes. To be honest, the kind of crowd I wished to have around me then was the one that encouraged me, not question me. My thoughts had by then taken me closer to the practical aspects.

Suppose I were to donate an organ, which other age, which other stage in my life would have suited me? So if not now, then when?

By then, a few months had passed since Valsa's death. Life and business matters were flooding up around me. Our inverters, fans and stabilizers were doing very well in the market. Wonderla, our water theme park was running smoothly. The charity under my father's trust was managed well at Thrissur. Sheela's garment business was also doing well. My sons were looking after our businesses. Arun and Priya were in Bengaluru. My younger son Mithun and his wife Joshna were in Kochi. I had stopped mentioning the possibility of kidney donation. Everyone around me thought I had dropped the idea.

Chapter 4

Finally, it Happens

When I came to Cochin thirty-three years ago, I only had a second-hand Lambretta scooter. My whole business was built up on that old blue scooter. Soon after, I joined the Rotary Club. There were a few of us friends in the club who had begun our lives in a similar modest manner. We were newly married, with supportive wives, small kids and big ambitions. We did not have too much money but our calling gave us courage. Our goals were shining ahead of us, beckoning constantly, and we were ready to work towards it day after day.

Slowly and naturally, we found success in our own ways. One of my friends in the club became a reputed chartered accountant; another a famous architect who ran his own firm and a third became a highly accomplished lawyer. We were a jolly bunch. They knew I always worked according to my plans and respected me. Those who knew me from such close quarters never questioned me.

Yet, when I started my ventures, I did face resistance from elsewhere. My choices were considered as mere fancies and my ideas were brutally questioned. Take the case of our water theme park in Ernakulam. When I thought of setting up a water amusement park in Kerala, some of my financial advisors and auditor friends gave it the thumbs down. They had an impressive array of statistics to prove how wrong my idea was. All those water theme parks in Hyderabad and Bombay (now Mumbai) had failed. They had the right figures to back up their arguments—the expenses, the revenues were all very telling. These gentlemen were correct from the point of view of these statistics. However I could see evidence of trouble in those papers. They conclusively argued that I should not launch the park.

However by then, my heart and head were set on this idea. All I could tell them was that I was neither a chartered accountant nor a holder of a business administration degree like them. I was a simple man with a simple idea that I thought people would love. Their reservations just couldn't dissuade me. We launched Veegaland water theme park in 2000 in Kochi. It was renamed Wonderla and continues to be a stunning success both in popularity and earnings.

Haven't we read in books that those who succeed need to pass through failures?

Achievers always try many things before finding their true calling and source of success. I often took calculated risks. They were based on my hunches and my own ways to measure a possibility. However, if I burnt my hand, I simply walked away. That was it. There were incidents in my life where I was grossly mistaken in my judgments and had retreated.

Unlike these business investments, this time, in the case of organ donation, the choice was about investing in myself. Thus my own reputation was at stake. My company's credibility rested on a certain amount of goodwill. I could not afford to let down my entire entrepreneurial establishment with a foolish choice. From the point of announcing the decision till it took place in a successful way, I wanted things to go right. It was a tall order. However I had a stern view that V-Guard was not to be known by the name of a Chairman who made a quixotic decision. My staff and the entire business network built around my previous decisions were not to be rocked by any mishap. It was not just a matter of my kidney. It was my entire life work itself that I was about to place on the platter.

Like many others, whenever I wanted to make a choice in life or business, I always did my own research about the issue. When V-Guard stabilizers were ready to be sent to the market, I was the only staff member in my company who could look after marketing as well. So every day I carried two boxes of three stabilizers each in both my arms and got into trains. Sometimes I went to northern Kerala, other times to southern areas, holding these boxes. I went to electronic shops and sold the stabilizers which I had manufactured myself. When I saw similar scenes in the movie *Pursuit of Happyness*, featuring Will Smith, I smiled because I, too, had been in a similar position once. Till I was sure others could contribute the way I wanted, I preferred to work on my own.

Once the kidney donation idea hit me, I wanted to know every bit of information before cementing my decision. I didn't surf the internet but I had a secretary who gladly did the same for me. He began sending me files named 'Kidney'. Day after day, my inbox began getting choked with mail attachments containing details about kidney and organ transplanting—both on donating and receiving. Somebody in the office took printouts for me, which I read in my free time.

This whole affair of giving away an organ and getting and fixing it in a body was a fascinating world of information. The possibility of organ transplantation was actually realized during the Second World War. When some soldiers came in with bullets in their kidney, doctors had to remove the entire damaged kidney and still those men lived for decades. That led medical science to contemplate the possibility of kidney donation to those with damaged kidneys.

Then they tried to transplant it. Initially they transplanted organs in identical twins and that was successful. Many say that the ancient surgeon Sushruta was the one who introduced the idea of surgical transplanting in India. And some in the medical fraternity believe Europeans followed this Indian idea later.

All of this was fascinating, but I had to be wary of the information I obtained from the internet. Anyone could come and feed information there—wrong or half-true. Nevertheless, such investigations are important when you have a focus. These enquiries are part of strengthening your vision. We do things well only by understanding them thoroughly. I had to tread with care by consulting a doctor on this. Not one. So I began calling several doctors I knew. Nothing about the subject would have bored me. Some of the willing doctors talked with me for hours whenever we got time. I was told that in modern times, the first experimental kidney and liver transplants were tried in dogs. Among the articles my secretary downloaded for me, I read about a certain Dr P.K. Sen and his team from King Edward VII Memorial Hospital in Mumbai who did this somewhere in the 1950s. I would have just been born then.

At home, after supper, I sat with the printouts, poring over them to learn more. In the same hospital in Bombay, they also did the first human kidney transplant surgery. This was in May 1965. I would have been fifteen years then. Next year, another surgery took place. Then another took place in Varanasi. I was curious about the results of these surgeries. The first patient died on the eleventh post-operative day. The second patient died on the third day after the operation. These were recipients who had taken the organs from dead bodies. Another report said that a successful live donor transplant in India happened six years after these operations—CMC

Hospital at Vellore did it this time. This was soon followed by several thousand transplants.

I wanted to get some kind of figures. No proper documentation was in place. Hence it was nearly impossible to get an exact number of transplants done so far in India. What we do know is that the medical fraternity in India has advanced greatly from that year of the first transplant. So much so that one can go back home the next day after the surgery and start a normal life in just two weeks. Still, *Kidney International*, the journal of the International Society of Nephrology, said India does only about 3, 200 transplants every year, although no one could confirm that as the precise figure.

If you were looking for reliable numbers, there was only one statistic that everyone agreed on; every year, India needs at least 150,000 kidneys!

Normally, donation happens when there's an emotional bond between the recipient and the donor. A spouse may give it to his or her partner, or a parent may give to the child. I knew a case in my town, where a person had donated his kidney to his family friend's daughter since the parents of the girl could not do so. So this man went ahead and gave it voluntarily. There was a palpable sense of charity on the part of the donor here, as also a strong element of affection in it. I still haven't exactly figured out which one of these impulses prompted me. I guess it could be a mixture of all these elements. For a mere sense of self-centred accomplishment or adventure, I wouldn't have let anyone place a knife on me. To feel the bliss of charity, I had already been doing enough. I knew that I need not have offered my body over and above it. As far as affection goes, I had no needy recipient in mind to offer after Valsa's death; no agonized face in particular in mind. Perhaps all these together in parts and pieces worked within me. At some point in life I stopped assessing what really prompts certain decisions in us.

In life, isn't it true that we don't get answers to a lot of questions? Why were we born in this shape, size and colour? Why do we have the parents we have? Why did we decide in favour of the vocation we chose? Why did we marry the woman or man we have now?

We'll never know for sure.

We might know more on the 'whats' and 'hows' of life, but not many of those 'whys' will be answered. So I let the matter rest in the question itself.

Any surgery means cutting through the layers of our body—its skin and flesh and reaching the inside of our body. It is a bloody sight if we see the video. My wife and sons haven't seen my surgery video yet. I have kept it away safely somewhere in the drawers.

The fact is that I was once someone who would faint at the sight of blood. I remember an instance: My younger brother was very good at sports. He was six years younger than me and I was like a guardian to him. I was the one who took him to school. When I was in the sixth standard and he was in the first, he fell while playing and his head bore a deep cut. My uncle rushed him to a hospital. Our father was elsewhere. I was there at the hospital—before the duty doctor dressed up the wound, we saw his skull, the inside of the scalp. I suddenly felt giddy. Somehow I grabbed on to the bench and saved myself from falling. The doctor, noticing my fright, asked me to go out and shut the door behind me. Meanwhile, my brother sat there with such ease, answering the doctor's questions.

I guess my later life with all the layers of experiences made a new being out of me. We mature like wine. At some point we even begin to lose the fear of death, I suppose. Some of us, at least.

A month later, with the thought growing and strengthening, I called up a nephrologist who was a friend of a friend. I raised the issue with him. By now, I was more or less sure that I was going to proceed with the donation. The elderly doctor, to whom I was still a stranger, scolded me.

'If you have so much of an "urge", buy a kidney for some poor fellow or a dialysis machine for some needy hospital. It'll only cost you around five lakh rupees.'

I realized it was meaningless discussing this matter with the gentleman. I needed a staunch supporter of my cause. I was getting impatient and fed up of such cynics and critics. I wanted an organ donation evangelist. Finally one day, I found the right person, perfect for the emotional, moral and technical support that I required to build my venture of donation.

When we embrace an idea or a subject, information or advocates of the same idea appear before our eyes, in the form of some news report or a television show or even as somebody's passing talk?

It happened to me too.

Around that week or the next, I chanced upon a news report about a priest named Fr Davis Chiramel who had donated his kidney. My brother John, living in Thrissur, told me that he had once met this priest. He got me Fr Chiramel's number. About a year ago Fr Chiramel had donated his kidney to a poor electrician who couldn't afford to buy one. Fr Chiramel's was a different kind of affection for his recipient. It came from a greater wish to stand by a weak man, to strengthen someone with one's own organ. The priest never knew the patient. When he heard the money gathered for the unfortunate man was not sufficient to pay for a kidney, Fr Chiramel simply said, 'Take mine'.

I learnt that there was another priest who donated his kidney to a boy who was his badminton partner. I wondered why such great acts do not become big news. We thirst for some other kind of news. However this was where life's greater drama lay. Greater than what comes out of the state assemblies or cricket stadia. Greater than what happens at political party offices. We truly need to look at such mighty acts of human will and learn important lessons.

Isn't this where the real acts of nation-building lay? More than even nation-building, don't such acts help us all evolve into greater human beings?

Let me return to Fr Chiramel's story.

A certain electrician lived in the same village as this priest. He was an earnest man; a simple and honest person with a loving family. He fell ill due to a weak kidney. Some youngsters set up a committee and Fr Chiramel was appointed as its head. They somehow managed to collect around two to three lakh rupees. But that was not enough for the surgery. They were short of another five lakhs. It was almost impossible to raise such a big sum from the village. In that committee meeting, Fr Chiramel stood up and said in that case, he would donate his kidney. It stunned everyone. And so it was that the age of forty-eight, Fr Chiramel brought a dying man back to life. Some small newspapers printed the news, one of which came into my hands.

I rang up the priest and introduced myself. He said that he had heard of me.

I told him, 'I called to tell you that you've overtaken me in this. I'd been carrying this wish for a while now. Congratulations. I am actually jealous of you.'

Fr Chiramel was taken aback. He mumbled some replies. I felt that he was totally sceptical of my phone call and my wish. Three days later, he came to meet me.

He came home and told me straight to my face. 'I want to know if you're serious about this.'

When the priest came home for the first time, Sheela had gone visiting our son and family in Bengaluru. Fr Chiramel could have had his share of doubts. No successful businessman had, to his knowledge, offered to donate his own organ before. He could well have thought that I was trying to create news headlines. He did not know me in person and since these days people go to any length to be in the news, he wanted to know how serious I was. I confirmed it and asked him to recommend me to a good doctor. Finally he was convinced. He now wanted to know where Sheela stood on this decision. He knew better than to ignore her opinion because in his experience 80 to 90 per cent of donor volunteers change their minds when their spouses put their foot down. Fr Chiramel told me that he had visited countless homes based on phone calls from people saying they were willing to donate their kidneys. However by the time he reached their homes, they would have changed their minds. He was expecting the same in my case too. I wanted to show him how serious I was and so I invited him again.

On Fr Chiramel's second visit, they both met. We were having breakfast. I was apprehensive and sat looking at Sheela. He spoke to her. Once Fr Chiramel decided that Sheela wasn't strongly opposed to the idea, he began elaborating on how comfortably he was living after donating one of his kidneys. He told us—rather her—he was more active after the donation. He had gone to Jerusalem and had visited three or four European countries. He established the Kidney Federation and was busy with its activities. In his kind way, he told Sheela that there was nothing to worry about. He stretched the hour of our breakfast so that he could elaborate on the advantages of organ donation. Sheela sat there, unsure and unhappy about the course of things. Like any wife, she was worried for me.

Later when we were together, I assured the good priest, 'Chances are slim that she would argue with you, Father.' We laughed in unison.

Upon my request for a good physician, Fr Chiramel suggested the name of Dr Aby Abraham of the Lakeshore Hospital. Fr Chiramel said the doctor was comparatively young. That gave me hope for I believed he would have more courage; that he'd be liberal enough to consider a sixty-year-old as a donor. I had known many physicians over the decades, but had not heard of him. Dr Aby had come to Lakeshore recently and was previously a nephrologist at the Vellore Medical College Hospital. Dr Aby was quite a sprightly guy and had overseen several donations. He worked along with Dr George who had done about 1,100 kidney transplant surgeries by then. That was a mind-boggling figure. So many surgeries, so many lives—admiration for this physician team grew in me. Usually the kidney is taken by opening the part where it is. However this doctor had specialized in laparoscopic surgery. It was a safer and easier route. Hence a lot more people came to him.

It was Dr Aby who had helped transplant Fr Chiramel's kidney. I requested Fr Chiramel to speak to him on my behalf. Every donation requires a series of medical tests to determine if the kidneys can be given and whether after donating, the body will remain stable. Fr Chiramel promised me he would check with Dr Aby. I began to get a feeling that I was nearing my destination. My heart felt lighter and I rejoiced. Fr Chiramel did constant follow-ups and kept calling me every day or the other to talk and to share his news. Slowly but surely, my wish began to flower.

Sheela was not fully convinced yet so she continued to voice her concerns. I began avoiding her questions by saying 'Let us do the tests first'. When her queries increased, I rephrased that statement into some kind of a retort.

'What's wrong in doing the tests?'

I was trying to douse the fire in her heart.

Chapter 5

At the Other End of the Rainbow

Finally, the day came for me to meet Dr Aby Abraham. He was much younger than I thought. The nephrologists I had taken advice from earlier had been older.

'Hope you are aware of my intention,' I told him.

He had already been briefed by Fr Chiramel. Dr Aby asked me if I was really serious; I said yes. He explained to me how a kidney functions and how a transplant is usually done. He said that one-third of a kidney was enough to keep a man healthy. If the function goes weaker, then he will need a transplant. One kidney, medical science says, can be dispensed with, if the other one is functioning well. That made me wonder why a human body would have an organ that is not absolutely necessary. Then I realized we have a second ear and a second eye and a pair of arms and legs, though only one of these would be enough for survival. Perhaps they are like spare parts.

Is our physiological system offering us a grand opportunity to be compassionate to a fellow being? Or does our body intuitively know that we would abuse our organs with our lifestyle and might need a spare part once in a while?

Then Dr Aby said they would have to do lot of tests on me. I said I was ready to undergo all these and I would pay for everything. All I wanted was to keep my anonymity; I told him I didn't want any special privilege or concession on the bills considering that I was there to donate a kidney. The good doctor smiled. He said to start off, he would recommend a few preliminary tests. If I passed them I'd be asked to undergo more tests. It felt like I was sitting for my graduation exams.

My series of tests began with blood and urine samples. I didn't know then that this was only the start of a very long journey.

Dr Aby explained to me about laparoscopic surgery. The technique allows people to donate a kidney with much less inconvenience. It requires a shorter hospital stay and the recovery is quicker. In this method, surgeons make a small incision at the navel, about two-and-a-half inches wide. They also make four small holes to insert instruments. The laparoscope has a miniature camera, which shows the inside of a body on a video monitor. Surgeons watch the video to disconnect the kidney with the inserted scissors. Once the kidney has been cut and the arteries clipped for good, it is wrapped in a plastic bag and taken out through the small incision at the navel. All done mechanically.

On the other hand, the traditional 'open' surgery needs a deep cut of about ten inches length. It cuts through abdominal muscles and takes a long time to heal. This old method of surgery left a long incision mark with stitches prominently displayed. On the other hand, the donors who choose the laparoscopic technique are asked to follow a post-surgical pain medication for an average of only twenty-seven hours. In the case of traditional surgery, this was sixty hours. However before all that I had to become a candidate for donation.

I sat there and saw several hurdles staring at me.

Every journey begins with a small step. But when we have only the destination in mind, and are eager to reach there, sometimes these small steps can appear frustrating, however much we know they are inevitable. In life, things take their due time. As there is a season to bear fruit, there is also a season to remain patient. This applies to any area of life and in entrepreneurship too. Patience and tenacity of purpose are two great tools to succeed in life.

When I was twenty-three, I boarded a bus from my village and came to Thiruvananthapuram to become a supervisor trainee for a monthly salary of ₹150. It was a small step. If I had been too eager in my mind to reach my present position, I would have got nervous and impatient. It took another thirty-seven years to come to this moment.

I began visiting the Lakeshore Hospital for my tests.

Some have shown surprise at my spending so many hours in queues to get tested and all the expenses I undertook. There were times while waiting in the queues when I wished I were somewhere else. I overcame such weaknesses of mind by repeating the same actions. I did such experiments upon myself to see how far I could go. I would push myself to see how far my limits could stretch—patience, willpower, goodwill, mental strength, tolerance, and so on. It definitely helps you to grow.

The secret of success is to push ourselves. We should do things that are good for us even if we don't feel like doing them. We should do them again and again till we overcome our inertia. That will take us to where we want to be. The first time, it will be hard. When we do it for the second time, our urge to quit will lessen. That's how we keep building our mind's stamina little by little.

It's easy to quit. If we quit, we lose. I draw energy from self-help books. I love reading positive, inspirational literature. I used to read novels when I was younger. Then I stopped reading fiction and switched over to self-improvement books. I also read biographies of eminent people and entrepreneurs. How these successful ones got there was of genuine interest to me. In college, I was a mediocre student. Most often, I just skimmed through the textbooks. However to win, we have to to learn about life itself to deal with challenges.

Lakeshore Hospital, where I was going for the tests, was run by eminent doctors. I was good friends with some of them.

Dr Aby said I would need clearances from all departments including cardiology, neurology, nephrology and psychiatry. On one of those customary visits for tests to the cardiology department, a charming nurse gave me a big broad smile. There was such affection in her, something I never expected in a hospital. She then told me she had once worked in one of my companies. That alarmed me. I was trying to remain anonymous here in the hospital. We exchanged pleasantries. I told her that there was nothing wrong with my health and this was just a routine check-up. I wanted to keep the whole process under wraps. However hospitals are big places where we can bump into anyone. I realized I had been naïve to think I could hide my plan.

The days of tests were not easy on me either. After a bunch of tests, when I thought it was getting over, another set came up. Some days I stood in queues with relatives of the patients to pay the bill. Most often someone recognized me. Each such instance made me nervous. Appearing for a test sometimes meant being on a fast and spending hours travelling up and down keeping away from every other engagement.

I'm a man who spends a lot of time in solitude at home. Some days I wished I were back in my room rather than in this hospital with all these strangers around me. I wished I were in my bed reading a book. I wished I were in office sitting and overseeing some happy growth factor in my company. There were so many better getaways than being in a hospital, I thought. However there wasn't any other way out. I had chosen this and now I had to go through it all. It was vexing yet I somehow stood my ground. I wanted to see where these tests were taking me and what kind of results awaited me. A sense of curiosity drove me on.

One day, I was asked to come for a new test quite unexpectedly. The doctor said my urine from twenty-four hours was to be monitored. I was handed over a large five-litre can in the lab. I was mortified. I didn't want anyone in the hospital to see me carrying this huge can. I begged the pharmacy man to give me some wrapper or cover to hide the can. I came out of the hospital, embarrassed and fearing some strangers would pop up and recognize me. All I wanted was to be back home right away. The can was wrapped and held under my arm. The next day I had to be at the office. So I took a plastic bottle with me and brought back what I urinated during my office hours. I saved the entire urine from those twenty-four hours—about three litres—and took it back to the hospital the next day. The same ordeal took place again and I had to hide it from everyone. People might think I was silly for making such a fuss. For some reason I didn't want to face any questions from anyone.

Certain tests demanded my repeated visits. Sometimes I had to come on another day to pick up the results. I had to be there in person since it included consultations with the doctors. Besides, I didn't want to drag anyone else into this process, however tiresome it was. Most often, these doctors had a large assembly of patients waiting at their doors. I'd wait among them and some, who recognized me would stare at me. The obvious queries being, 'What happened? or 'What's wrong?'

Whenever possible, the doctor would ask his attending nurse to bring me in, knowing I was there on a mission. I had made it clear I wanted no preference. Yet some always made way for me. It was an act of kindness and I accepted it gracefully. Yet, what I found embarrassing was answering questions of some doctors or attendants like, 'Is something wrong with you?'

I'd try and tell them that this was to avoid surprises, to know my state of health. However then a little later most of them would know that the tests were not just for that. Then the obvious question would be 'Why?' I'd smile and try to brush it away. However doctors being doctors, they insisted on getting answers. When I found myself surrounded by junior doctors, most of them recognizing me, I would begin to get nervous.

My prominent worry was the possibility of a rejection by the hospital for medical reasons.

Finally one day Dr Aby rang me up and said I had passed all the tests. It was like topping my graduation exams, but my jubilation died quickly.

Dr Aby added, 'But since you are sixty and a public persona, I'm afraid we'll have to put you through more tests to doubly ensure that we are making the right move.'

It made sense, although it was also bitter to think of doing things over again. I had to swallow it.

'Okay', I mumbled.

I had a personal task to do before that—letting my family know. Till then, when close friends or relatives had asked, I'd skim over the topic. I had thought I needn't convince anyone of the merits and demerits of my decisions. I was an independent man. When V-Guard was running smoothly, I had jumped into launching Veegaland. I could not sit pretty on my achievements and even now, I'll keep searching for the right opportunities to fulfil the wish, the vision. I needed to keep raising the bar. My decision to donate was clearly based on my reasoning too, knowing that this was such a conducive time for donating. If my parents were alive and had opposed me, I wouldn't have done this. If my children were young and relying on me for their survival, I would have backed out. If a little son or daughter had pulled on my sleeve, begging me not to be adventurous, I'd have succumbed to their plea. If my health was poor, I would have anyway ruled this out. Our views change as we grow older.

If I were thirty or forty, I might not have done it. Indian thought prescribes an age for doing things in a systematic way; Brahmacharya, Grihsthashrama, Vanaprastha, Sanyasa. How right those sages were! A grihastha wouldn't be able to do things at his free will. He can earn his freedom to do so only after completing his karma or fulfilling his responsibilities towards his family. It was somehow all favourable to me. However I did not feel like explaining all this back then to my relatives or inquisitive friends.

Besides all those tests, I was also required to go get some more tests done from agencies outside. What they wanted to know was if both my kidneys were working perfectly. By then I had visited the hospital at least a dozen times in just over a month. Back home, in a diary, I wrote down all the dates of my visits. That week, my next series of tests began. I went to a scanning centre attached to the Lourdes Hospital. Both my kidneys had to be in perfectly healthy condition and had to be sharing the functions equally. If one was weak, I would be rejected. I got nervous again.

I had to reveal my purpose again at the hospital. The physician in charge stared at me and then went back to the papers. He began looking through them once again earnestly. It was with much anxiety that I told him my wish. I found myself overcome by a sense of shame while revealing it. I wondered if he would think I was aiming too high, for too big a plan, while not having the required health. I held a shy smile to cover my embarrassment. Mine was a villager's timidity; as if I were asking for something I did not deserve. A couple of days later I was called back. The physician kindly told me that both my kidneys were just fine and functioning as required for the purpose. He congratulated me and wished me good luck. Something welled up in me. I nodded at him happily. I had passed yet another examination.

Then came the day to visit the psychiatrist at the hospital. Dr Aby was a bit hesitant to inform me that it was mandatory on a donor's part to pay the psychiatrist a visit. It was to medically assess that the donor was making a decision with a sound and healthy mind. In these parts of the world, to pay a visit to a psychiatrist had a surprisingly damaging effect on the image of the person. It affects us poorly to imagine that we need psychological support but the world is changing. The stigma attached to such practices also will go some day. Anyway, this explains why Dr Aby was hesitant. He said it was a formality as they needed all papers duly signed in the file. I had no problem with this test whatsoever. If they needed to know that my mind is sound, then I would go and present myself.

The psychiatrist was more business-like. He said he wanted to understand the rationale of my decision. When I sat before him I felt he was being plain and matter-of-fact. Perhaps that was why I felt he was questioning me like a policeman and for a moment, I felt like a suspect. In the next moment, I knew this was a routine question. He asked me why I had decided to donate my kidney. I didn't feel like explaining it then so I mumbled some vague reason. I was further asked if I slept well, ate well and if I was under stress. I answered satisfactorily, but I was not sure that these answers of mine satisfied him.

The gentleman came closer to me and asked, 'Do you have any other problem?'

I couldn't hold back my chuckle.

'I guess my problem is that I don't have any problem.'

It didn't seem to make any impression on him. The psychiatrist kept staring into my eyes as if trying to find some fault. Maybe I was nervous. Maybe I wanted it all to end. It's human sometimes to get fed up. However like always, I drew my mind back again to the drawing board, telling myself, I had come this far. Now it was a matter of a few days till I got the final results.

The very next day, while I was in my office looking through some business papers, Dr Aby rang up.

'Hearty congratulations, Sir, let me officially break the news: you are medically fit to donate a kidney,' he said.

That was the big moment.

I felt a wave of joy filling me. Finally, after all those long trials and tests and worrisome nights and days and all those boring trips back and forth to the hospital, after all those countless conversations and questions and answers, after all those hesitations and fears of others', my single wish had stood ground and flowered. I could donate a kidney to anyone I wished. It was like getting a fat bank account to write a hefty cheque. I felt vindicated. Tears welled up in my eyes. I didn't know why.

Then, I remembered a strange fact. I had written an article—my first—when I was nineteen and a second year B.Sc student at St Thomas College. I had written a commentary about the first heart transplant in the world that happened around that period. My piece was a satirical take on an imaginary brain transplant. A friend had read it and taken it to the college magazine editor who published it that year. It surprised me now that the first article I ever wrote was about organ donation and after forty-one years, I was granted a wish to donate a vital organ. I think, in some strange ways, we carry seeds of certain thoughts right from birth or childhood. I don't know. I just wondered what on earth made me write such a piece even when I was young and naïve. Now here I was, ready to deliver!

Only I knew the truth.

Chapter 6

Quakes and Quivers

To this day, I am still surprised by the reactions and responses of the people around me to the donation of my kidney. Many could not understand me. I don't know if they tried to do so without prejudice.

My surprise springs from two facts. One, by the sheer number of discussions this decision evoked around me. I had never intended or had a clue that my wish would occupy so much space and time in the media as well as in the conversations of people in various towns and villages. I had thought the earnestness of my wish would be appreciated. I don't look for such appreciation; but as a social being I knew this was would come whether I intended it or not.

The second thing that took me aback were the varied and contrasting ways of responding to or looking at the idea. I had merely thought of it as an act of goodness. I never imagined some people, who did not even know me in person, could turn it around into a story of hate. It was a big life lesson.

But first, I had to stay tough to face questions from my family. It was never going to be easy. Each member had a different way of looking at it and was deeply emotionally involved. I kept thinking how I would face Sheela's questions. I didn't want to hurt her or anyone for that matter. Neither did I want my wish to be blown out of proportion. However, I also quickly realized that if I were to mellow down and start using my time to cajole and pacify each member, I would lose a lot of energy and they'd overpower me emotionally. I knew it would be impossible to convince Sheela. The truth is, I did not make an effort, which the task demanded.

I told her, 'I don't expect you to give me a "go ahead" because I know and respect your concerns about me. But that doesn't mean my decision will change.'

I had pencilled in a cut-off date in my mind.

I was to turn sixty on 27 December. I had decided that I would go ahead with the procedure right after my birthday. Sheela, who first thought my wish was a joke or a passing fancy, was shocked to learn that the donation was finally happening. She began to worry obsessively about the result of the surgery and objected vehemently to it. My children and their spouses began to wonder what was going on in my head. To a large extent, Priya spoke in favour of me. Obviously, memories of her mother's illness were still fresh in her mind.

She didn't directly encourage me though.

Instead, she said, 'I too will definitely donate in the future.'

Sheela was not as vociferous in her objections on hearing this. Arun too took a neutral stance after a while. They had done their research and concluded that I wasn't totally out of my senses. They knew that a lot of people donate their kidneys and there was nothing unusual about it. The donors were living without any health problem. They were not only physically fit but also satisfied that they had saved a life.

Mithun also gave it a lot of thought and tried to understand it from the scientific point of view. Yet, my sons were apprehensive since it was none other than their father who was involved. They tried to dissuade me by saying that although I was not wrong in my decision, there wasn't any urgent need for such a donation now. I sensed how intelligent they were. They knew well I wouldn't budge a bit even if they opposed me. So they were trying their best to diffuse the heat in me. I felt their love for me. In fact, I felt it in many different ways.

All those responses, given their varied nature—some vehement, some angry, some hurt, some trying to cajole—told me more about what they felt for me. I would be lying if I said wasn't touched by it all. I was touched that Sheela was so worried about me. I didn't express my feelings and how much I was moved by their responses. I wrapped it all inside and went about getting the medical tests done.

Call it my way of loving them back.

A venerable physician advised me to donate money for ten kidney transplant operations since I was so passionate about the cause. I asked him whether it could equal what I wanted to do. He fell silent. In what I was about to do, there was real action. We don't give from what has come to us, like money or goods. We give what's ours. I was confident that nothing untoward would happen to me. It was an intuition—my deeper mind told me to go ahead.

I also had a counter-argument that even if something bad happened to me, I wouldn't let the worry affect me. My family was well taken care of. My sons were married. My wife was contented with the life we had made together. There were no financial worries. I wanted to do something meaningful with my life and in reaching this decision I had found an amount of peace, certainty and confidence in life itself. Deep within, I was sure that I wasn't going to die on the surgery table.

Over the months when I had thought about it, I was clear about one thing. My act was not charity. I used to tell Fr Chiramel that I was just giving away an old kidney. It was a joke between us.

For me it was not an act of largeheartedness. Maybe it was more like an adventure. I wanted the public to know that there is no harm in giving away a kidney; to let the world know that no amount of money spent on advertising could achieve as much awareness about organ donation as this act could. Only such action could convince the populace. But it was Fr Chiramel who turned it into a social cause by putting my kidney at the head of a donation chain. That's a story which will come later.

On the day Dr Aby called to break the good news to me, I came home at noon and stood in the living room with a big smile. I saw Sheela staring at me. I told her that I was medically fit at the age of sixty to donate a kidney. Sheela turned pale. Along with Arun and Mithun, she was secretly hoping that I would somehow get rejected medically. Sheela went away and sat alone. This was really a torturous moment for her. He who takes the decision needs to go through the fear just once—at that moment of his decision. After that, it's a game for him. But his dear ones need to bear and watch with no control over the decision and it's pretty hard. They are the ones who should be supported. In the case of Sheela, I must say I did not go beyond a point to convince or cajole. I knew it would not have worked. Before the result had come, whenever we were alone, Sheela would sit worried and I would go and try to cheer her up. I would tell her that now we were well settled, and our children were happy and my parents were no more.

Then she would look at me painfully and ask, 'What about me then? Don't you care about me?'

I would somehow try to pacify her. I knew I failed every time I tried convincing her. All I could do was hope that when everything was over, she would see it was the right decision.

My sense of jubilation grew as my sixtieth birthday came closer. I rang up Fr Chiramel and broke the news. I asked him to round up eligible candidates and then zero in on the right one. Although I had decided to donate my kidney, I had no recipient in mind. I thought it would be better if the person was financially needy.

I also thought maybe it would be better if the person were not a Christian. We live in a strange society. Our acts and thoughts are interpreted in an odd way here. Some would read a communal angle into this. Since the two persons involved, Fr Chiramel and I, were Christians, we thought it would be best to pass it on to someone from a different religious background. This should not be turned into some parochial community affair.

The gesture had to have a true resonance of love in it. That was our position. I told Fr Chiramel that I was not concerned who the recipient was. If one could call it a condition, I had only one: The recipient should be a poor person whose kidney had failed owing to natural causes and not due to a reckless life. I wanted to pacify myself that the pains I had taken were to be reciprocated by a recipient who truly deserved it.

It wasn't even necessary that I come into contact with the person. I had no problem if the person and I didn't even meet. I wasn't looking for anyone to fall at my feet out of gratitude. The truth is, when it all started, I had actually wanted to keep it all anonymous. I would have been happier if it were done without a single soul other than the doctors knowing that I was the donor. I would have happily lived with such anonymity.

But the world around me had other plans.

Finding the recipient was Fr Chiramel's task. He was running a kidney donor organization and was in touch with several parishes in Kerala. They were always on the lookout for the right person. One day, Fr Chiramel informed me that he had identified the recipient of my kidney. I said I didn't want to know anything about him. My feeling then was to donate the organ and disappear. I didn't want anything to do with the recipient, let alone a bonding. It was then that Fr Chiramel told me about this strange idea of his.

He had a plan.

Soon after he had donated his own kidney, Fr Chiramel had realized that the country had numerous kidney patients who needed immediate attention. One factor that defeated those helpless patients was the legal hazards they had to face. These include unnecessary bureaucratic hurdles, intimidating attention from the police and other authorities, exorbitant medical expenses, and finally, an extreme scarcity of healthy kidneys. Fr Chiramel thus decided this was the best moment to start a chain of donation in the state. He was actually waiting for a voluntary donor to start his plan.

A person voluntarily donates his or her kidney. One of the recipient's family members volunteers in return to donate to another needy person and the chain goes on.

Fr Chiramel said, 'If the guy we choose is ready and medically fit to receive the organ, I'll ask his wife or any close relative to donate a kidney to a needy and matching patient. That patient's relative or family members should donate to another and so forth.'

It appeared like a meaningful plan.

'Your kidney should start a chain of grace and many lives will be saved with no money coming in between,' he said.

The priest began his calculation and said this way it could grow into a mighty donor movement. I did not jump onto the bandwagon immediately. I warned him if that one person breaks the vow, the chain would be broken. Yet it was worth trying. Besides, after Valsa's experience and my own meagre experience in these last few months learning about organ donation, I too was convinced that something good and large should come out of such a wish. So when the priest said he would donate my kidney to only such a person, I agreed.

Now, the time had come for me to break the news to my relatives. Coming to know about it from other sources would have hurt them. So I rang them up and disclosed my decision to donate a kidney. I told them that Fr Chiramel was looking for a recipient. When a family meet came up, I broke the news in person. My eldest sister, Sr Susheela, whom I call *Pengal* (Malayalam term for sister) is in the Apostolic Carmel convent in Kenya. Another sister, Sr Ancilla, was the principal of the Providence College in Calicut. Achamma, another sister, and John, my brother, were present as well. It was a rare get-together. Whenever my siblings who lived abroad came home, we gathered at my brother's house or mine.

That day, when I broke the news, everyone was stunned.

As expected, every single one of them vehemently disagreed, and it suddenly caused a wedge among us. We were like two valleys now, parted by the mountain of my idea. I was alone on one side. On the other side, all my beloved siblings and relatives opposed me fearing for my life and health. I saw pain on their faces when they questioned the rationale of my decision. Since our parents had gone from our world, we only had each other to hold on to. My choice of such a path shocked and pained them.

I understood their feelings but still stood my ground. Now that my sons too were are settled, it was time to prove my mettle. I wanted to tell those around me that my quest in life wasn't merely for money, that there are greater elements in life other than money.

My eldest sister forgot for a moment her venerable position in the Church and in the family and blurted out, 'Are you mad?'

Unlike the others, whom I dealt with using rejoinders or jokes or anecdotes, she wasn't an easy nut to crack. I could see where her anxiety was coming from.

Our younger brother had had a mild heart problem. He had been living in Kochi, the same town where I lived. One day he was hospitalized and died suddenly of a heart attack. It was a shock to us. *Pengal* was clearly worried she would lose another one of her remaining two brothers.

They all realized that I was determined to go through with this. That must have weakened them. I can only figure out how desperate each of them in the room might have been.

A few days later, when she had returned to Nairobi, *Pengal* called me and told me loud and clear, 'All I have are my two young brothers. And if you start acting like this, how can your *Pengal* sit this far in peace?'

I fell silent and tried to laugh. I tried belittling her fears. It didn't work. Then I had to use the moral stick. She was the elder one and knew me better than anyone else.

'You are a senior nun, a bride of Jesus. You should encourage me.'

I was chuckling inside, certain that she would fall for it, on the telephone I heard a pause. She sighed at the other end, 'If it were a few years ago, I'd have supported you. Now, at this age it's hard for me'.

I could understand. No one would like to send their loved one to a surgery table. She still requested me to call it off. When nothing worked, I told her to talk to my doctor who would assure her about the safety of the procedure. She finally relented.

The truth was, if she had talked with him and had he been frank, my plan would have gone awry. I was lucky she was assured by this trick of mine. Her calls never subsided though. I could see how terribly upset she was. God knows how many special prayer sessions she must have undertaken in her Nairobi monastic room for me till she heard I was safe.

Chapter 7

The Recipient

One day, I got a call from Fr Chiramel saying the person he had identified as the recipient was a match for the donation.

The patient had convinced his thirty-eight year-old wife to donate her kidney to form a chain. We were happy. But our happiness had a quick death. A few days later Fr Chiramel called to say that the person had 'slipped' away.

The reason was strange and funny.

Apparently, when some well-wishers of the potential recipient heard that the donor was sixty they vehemently opposed the idea. They explained to him that giving away his wife's 'young' kidney for a sixty-year-old kidney was a foolish idea. The man fell for that logic. He and his wife backed out. I hope the man finally found a kidney good enough for him. Because by waiting for a 'young' kidney, he only lost precious time.

Fr Chiramel began another frantic search for the right recipient.

Within a week, he called to inform me about another candidate whose name was Joy from Pala. Fr Chiramel went to meet his family. Joy was struggling to make both ends meet. He was a truck driver and had a failing kidney. The poor man had been carrying it for long since he had no money to replace it. Joy and his wife Jolly had been going from pillar to post to gather funds. Sympathetic villagers had raised some money for his treatment but that wasn't enough for a kidney transplant. Joy had to keep travelling by bus from his native Pala to Kottayam Medical College for his treatment. He had nearly stopped going for dialysis due to lack of money and was getting weaker. Hope was rapidly dimming for him.

Fr Chiramel saw the man's despair and told Joy that he would arrange a kidney at no cost. Joy and his wife were overwhelmed. Their tearful outburst of joy was understandable, given the near impossibility of getting a kidney for free in our country. Fr Chiramel had also informed the couple about the only condition: someone from his side should donate a kidney to another needy patient. Jolly agreed readily. The moment I heard about Joy's plight, I thought his was a deserving case. Fr Chiramel and I kept talking late into that night. Our mission was now making sense to us. We felt a kind of peace growing in our hearts. However, it was still too early to celebrate. The first step was to evaluate whether our blood types matched.

After consulting with me Fr Chiramel brought Joy to Ernakulam and rented a house for the couple and put him under Dr Aby's treatment. All the tests were conducted, including tissue matching. Our blood groups matched. Then came the tissue cross-matching. Donor and recipient matching are of three types: blood type matching, tissue type matching and cross matching. Each is distinct and important. Blood group matching is important in transfusions and it is equally important in kidney transplants. Another factor is the Rh factor, which is not part of the kidney, as it relates only to a particular cell type in the blood. It is important when it comes to blood transfusion.

Tissue matching is all about the genetic matching between donors and recipients. We all carry various genes, which give us our individuality. They determine features like blood and tissue proteins, which are unique to individuals. These proteins are called antigens and can be defined in blood tests. The compatibility aspect of these antigens decides if a donor's kidney will suit a particular recipient. After a series of such tests that lasted for three to four weeks, we heard from the hospital that Joy's body could accept my kidney.

Then another problem cropped up. A week later, we learnt that the doctors had detected a growth in Joy's body. The doctors said it was not a good sign. His blood samples were taken and sent for biopsy. We were asked to wait for the results, and depending on the results we would know if the growth was dangerous for him.

I began to think of this man to whom my kidney would go. Isn't life like a rainbow connecting people in special ways? Two souls meet for several reasons. Yet, the connection is impossible to ignore. Even if we decide to sit at home, without any social connections, somehow, we'll eventually get into some ties with somebody. It could be a doctor, a client, a co-passenger, a milkman, a neighbour in urgent need, or a stranger dialling a wrong number.

I thought of Joy many times since Fr Chiramel brought up his case. It wasn't easy to find the right man to offer a kidney free of cost. Once the candidate was found, the tests were to be cleared. Even after all that, the surgeries, both on the donor and the recipient had to be successfully performed. There were so many hurdles. Yet I thought of this truck driver and wondered what connected us. There was practically nothing that would have brought us together in the normal course of life. Mine was a choice rooted in my sense of accomplishment and deliverance of a deed, in a sense of adventure, and maybe a little bit of compassion.

And there was this man in another part of my state who drove trucks and found his organ failing. That man and his wife must have spent many anxious nights and days. They had worried where the money for the procedure would come from. They must have prayed a lot. And one fine day Fr Chiramel had visited them to announce he'd arrange a kidney for free.

Imagine the incredulous looks on their faces when they heard it! And how did Fr Chiramel connect with me?

What strange web connects us all without our knowing? Now I could only hope that the growth found in Joy's body would prove harmless and that we both would remain alive and safe through it all.

Meanwhile, I was also getting a bit impatient. I wanted this to be done and get on with my life. Fr Chiramel, on his part, was sure about the truth of the mission this time. He said he would not allow the kidney donation chain to be broken. He had sketched out a chart of donors. I looked at the chart. The pen and pencil marks showed a circle of lines and a few names. My kidney was to go to Joy, and his wife's to a lady. Her husband Sainuddin would be giving his to a certain John and John's mother to another person, and so on.

It was amazing—a beautiful idea weaving in some innocent souls and forming an unending chain. All these donors were found and chosen by Fr Chiramel. The chart looked impressive and Fr Chiramel sat in front of me flushed with excitement. As I sat there in our verandah, listening to his plan I knew that something good was going to happen.

But it all depended on Joy's biopsy results. If the tests were positive for some malignancy, our plans would collapse. Fr Chiramel became crestfallen at the very thought. I cheered him up with a few words and some warm tea. Two people, perfect strangers to each other a few weeks ago, sat together to plot something grand they had never thought about before.

That's the way life worked. It threw new ideas and adventures on our path every day. It was a matter of picking and choosing what you wanted.

Chapter 8

Crossing the River

One day in the middle of it all, I turned sixty.

The time to donate had arrived. By then, some of the committee members of Fr Chiramel's parish had come to know about our plan. Fr Chiramel was forced to seek their approval. The news began leaking out. Then one by one, my distant relatives started calling me. I sensed I couldn't keep the whole thing under wraps anymore. We had to announce it.

At the same time, I worried about how to declare the news without having gone through the procedure yet. My sense of caution made me want to tread slow and steady. I was facing some kind of uncertainty here. I wanted to make this venture successful and only then let others know. However Fr Chiramel called me one day and said he wanted a press conference right away. He sounded like he was on the edge. I was shocked and turned pale on the other end of the phone.

My strategy has always been to declare things only when I am 100 per cent sure of it happening. Else, I always keep my mouth shut. For me, it is a shame to retreat from a decision I have declared out in the open. I always try my best to fulfill my commitments. My close friends and business partners know this. It is never my habit to boast about my plans. I disclose just about 10 per cent of my plans. Once I implement and make them successful and then I make them public. But here, this good man in his white habit was determined and I had to stand by him. I wondered why he couldn't wait for the operation.

Fr Chiramel had two reasons. One, he feared the news would fizz off if it leaked out in bits. He wanted the news to come out in the form of a big public message from this deed. Only a well-arranged and well-attended press conference could help the story to come out in the entire state, he argued. Two, he had promised all these families waiting for the transplant, that he would meet the expenses. Only an official and collective declaration about this mission would help raise funds for the hapless ones.

However, I wasn't sure.

Eventually, we decided to address the media and go to the public with our plans. What remained to be known was the medical fitness of the recipient. Fr Chiramel was worried that if Joy's biopsy was negative, he would have to begin all over again and find another candidate. Till then his idea of the chain donation would have to be kept frozen. I shared his worries. FrChiramel kept calling me every day to update me on these issues. Each time when everything seemed to fall in place, there came a new hurdle.

Life's like that. We simply have to go through it all.

Chapter 9

The Clouds Clear

Joy's results finally came. They were positive. His growth was declared harmless. He was suitable to receive my kidney. An overwhelmed Fr Chiramel asked me if I could actively get involved in the activities of the Kidney Federation. I informed him that this donation would be my activity. He understood and valued my decision. We announced a press conference in Kochi in January 2011. Although we announced the press meet, I was apprehensive whether such a propaganda preceding the surgery would create unwanted publicity.

What if this did not happen properly after declaring it? What if one of us passed away before the donation took place? What if someone from outside torpedoed it using dirty tricks? What if the patient faced some last minute complication? Won't it all turn my wish to donate an organ into a public fiasco?

Fr Chiramel wouldn't buy any of these. He strongly opposed my objections with one simple and powerful logic.

He said, 'What if one evening a reporter got wind of it when you approach the police commissioner or the village officer for the official permission?'

He was right. The news would have leaked out in an undesirable manner. Fr Chiramel insisted that we hold a meet and declare it. This way the idea of donation will get the much desired impact. It would garner public support, the mission will get wider acceptance and his organization would get the much needed support.

On the day, I was a bit late in reaching the venue of the press meet. Before we went in, Fr Chiramel whispered to me that Joy was sitting in the crowd in the last row.

I saw him. He was a stout six-foot man with a healthy body and a thick moustache, but a bandage was visible on his hand. It was a port to take the needle inside for dialysis. That was the only visible sign of him being a patient. Otherwise Joy looked able and healthy. I realized then how deceptive looks could be.

I finally went up to him and spoke with him. No one from the media knew then that he was the recipient. Thus we could have a private meeting in a different room. Understandably, Joy and Jolly were quite emotional and told me at first they couldn't believe this was happening. Jolly almost broke down. I wanted to understate the level of emotion and told them that she too was donating and there was no need of any obligation.

I'd been very clear from the beginning that I was at no point going to bond with the recipient or anyone related to this affair. The last thing I wanted was anyone feeling grateful.

Our press meet was a complete success.

The journalists were wide-eyed. They just couldn't believe at first that the Chairman of V-Guard was going to donate his kidney to somebody with no blood or emotional connection. Most papers took it to page one. Television channels too had a field day.

The news got picked up by the national media too. Telephone messages, tweets, Facebook statuses, blog posts and emails spread all across Kerala and to other parts of the country. I graced magazine covers. There was an avalanche of news stories. To be honest, I never thought it would become so big. Two days after the press conference, one of the largest dailies in the country, *Malayala Manorama* wrote an editorial supporting the idea of donation. There was a three-week gap between the press meet and surgery. The day after the press conference, when the media had flashed the news, the battery of my mobile phone died by noon. That was when I fully understood the impact of my decision. I never imagined it would move people in such large numbers.

We had called the press meet not to drum up our glory but for practical reasons. Two kinds of responses erupt to any action or opinion. Likewise, my decision to donate an organ also created staunch enemies. It's funny to think of all that from this distance in time. I never expected anyone could find fault with my action. I thought any sensible person would see only good sense in it.

These opponents made me wonder about the perverseness of the human mind. They failed to discourage me though Fr Chiramel was deeply hurt. This amount of negativity was something he didn't expect. A friend of mine rang me up from Thiruvananthapuram and informed me about a leader from the Left party who derided me in a public speech. The leader had accused me for donating my kidney for cheap publicity. According to him, I had ulterior motives and I would not actually give away my kidney. I would get admitted in the hospital and buy a kidney from someone and donate it in my name. He said rich people like me could afford such tricks. I told my friend that we can't blame the man. His thoughts reflected the way he acted. Fr Chiramel, however, got upset. He wondered how people could dump their garbage on what we were doing. I laughed.

'It's not just me, they are slandering you too!'

We both broke into a hearty laugh. Laughter alone was the best reaction to such petty talk.

We didn't have time to lose.

As soon as the news spread, responses from my business partners, directors, friends, shareholders, auditors, government officials and office team leaders began flowing. Some of these were quite amusing. Soon after the declaration, a couple of junior managers came up to me.

'Sir, if you are doing this because of the commitment you

made, we've found a solution for you. Some of us discussed this thoroughly here and have decided that one of us will donate so that you needn't.'

I smiled. I was even perplexed why anyone should want to take my place on a surgery table. I declined their offer and said I would be back in three weeks.

To lighten the gravity of the situation, I raised logic.

'Didn't I go to Alaska last year? You had this place to yourself for four weeks. This time, it will be only three weeks.'

That was not an answer to their question. They didn't quite digest it, yet they remained silent. Senior managers kept asking at intervals whether I had any second thoughts. A certain senior manager called me up and advised me to not go ahead with the plan as his wife with whom I hadn't spoken before, and who had kept her safe distance till then in reference, was so upset that she had lost sleep thinking of my operation. I had to laugh.

'Even Sheela is sleeping well at my home, then what is wrong with your wife?'

Both were older than me and their concern was genuine. So I chose to explain the situation to them. I rang her up and reassured her.

I would be lying if I said there was no sense of pleasure in my decision to donate a kidney. Strange as it may sound, that was the truth. I did indeed find some pleasure in doing this.

Pengal asked me, 'Is this charity or an adventure?'

I said, '*Pengal*, it's a bit of both.'

To some it might sound a bit strange. However this is the reason to many, I'm a strange kind of man.

What do I think of myself? Oh, I like me very much.

When I came to Kochi with a wish to make a good stabilizer, all I had was the ₹1,00,000 I'd borrowed from my farmer father. I had promised to return the amount when I made some money. He had trusted me. I lived in a cheap lodge called Abdurahiman Lodge. My room had two single-size bare wooden beds. I slept on one and on the other I placed my soldering iron, testers, spare wires, batteries, IC and a few other materials that I had bought from the market. That bare bed was my research space. I was young and ambitious. I did not know a lot about the market. All I knew was that I could make a stabilizer that would cut off when the voltage fell or rose. The stabilizers made by big companies available in the market had no such facility. I also believed I could create a better-looking stabilizer. Every night I went out and ate at some wayside stall and then returned to my room to work on my stabilizer. In a few weeks I had developed my product. I went to an ironsmith and gave him my design for a stabilizer box; it had curves and slants that made it look a little better than the soap box stabilizer shapes then available. Then I went and bought some orange paint and painted it myself.

I was a loner but with a clear intention. What was born in that cheap lodge room became a ₹1750 crore national establishment with a decent presence in global markets in a few years. All we need is a simple faith in our mission. We don't need sycophants around us. That will only drain our energy and take away our focus.

There is a simple proposition I make with life and those around me. It's 'give and take respect'. I neither demand that others obey me nor do I take another's arrogance in silence. Even at home this was what I taught my sons—they give me my space, I will give theirs. Being in the news did upset some of my schedules, but being in the news wasn't entirely new to me. Neither was I new to speaking up about matters of public concern.

Chapter 10

Speaking Out

In 1998, when I was forty-eight years old, I had made a legal plea to legalize passive euthanasia. Euthanasia means painless killing of a patient suffering from some incurable or painful disease or in an irreversible coma. The practice, also known as 'mercy killing', is illegal in most countries. My plea back then was I should be allowed a natural death with only painkillers being administered to reduce the suffering, in case I'm afflicted by a terminal disease after the age of seventy.

However, the Indian judicial and administrative system did not have any provision to register my document prepared in this regard. I filed a case in the Ernakulam Sub Court. My plea was to offer the patient a choice in accepting or rejecting the treatment administered by doctors. I had argued that I must be given the right to refrain from accepting any treatment or medicines, if I chose to under such circumstances.

Like the thought about kidney donation, this was also a sudden idea. The chief trigger was again a case I had to witness. She was my aunt, my father's elder brother's wife who we called Valiamma. She was quite healthy and led a happy life. My uncle had passed away earlier. After his death, she was healthy enough to take care of herself. When she was around eighty-seven, she came to her daughter's home at Edappally where she fell down and fractured her thigh bone. I had visited her in the hospital, and the doctors had suggested a surgery. My aunt was against it, but her children, themselves around sixty or above, insisted on a surgery. As feared, the worst happened. A post-surgery wound refused to heal and she lay clenching fists and biting teeth, suffering all the pain.

Back when we were young, we had lived like an extended family though in different houses. There were walls in the front courtyard that divided our houses. But all of us lived in the same compound. To me, she was second only to my mother. She lay in the hospital room with several tubes running in and out of her body—a tube to pass urine and a tube to feed her through the nose and then an oxygen mask to help her breathe. In short, she was on a life support system.

When I sat there, looking at her, besides my pain for her, a terror grew in me. What if I met with such an accident, I feared this would be my state too. I shuddered at this thought. I wanted a noble life and a painless death. I did not want such a ceremonious medically assisted existence. I felt agony seeing her suffer like this. My poor aunt went through all that pain for twenty-two days before she died. I have always reasoned that her death showed her more mercy.

Make no mistake, I have great regard for the medical fraternity; for their diligence, dedication and immense contribution to the wellbeing of people. I am also aware that the longevity of human lives has increased considerably after the advent of modern medical treatments and a support system. But isn't it still a fact that medical science can help only in extending the existence of people suffering from a terminal disease or a near-fatal accident? My desire was to shorten the duration of suffering of such patients.

It was at that time I came to know that if one went on a fast and refused food or drink, one could be forcefully taken to hospital by the authorities. Since suicide is considered a crime, a case could be registered against those who choose to fast to death for attempting passive suicide. This meant I didn't have any rights on my life or body. I had wanted to plan my future so that I would not become a burden to my family in my old age. Like we plan your life, our insurance, our children's education and our business, we must also plan our old age. This is called geriatric planning.

I didn't want to be a helpless patient fed through tubes and kept alive for the sake of living. I'm certain that many such patients will speak against such artificial prolongation of life. Such means are in most cases used without the person's consent. It is a fact that many illegal, immoral and inhuman practices are resorted to by medical professionals for the sake of profit. Human life is a gift of nature. It is a sacred contract between an individual and nature. Every person is endowed with a bundle of natural gifts. The State may regulate the lives of people in the interest of common good, without stifling their rights. However life is a personal property of an individual over which no one else—including the State—has any absolute authority.

After moving the court, I began getting countless phone calls, including from national dailies. Wherever I went, the media came seeking my quotes. I believe I caused a sensation though I had no such intentions. Needless to say the incident gave birth to a big debate. I was invited to many forums to talk about this. Some of the forums I got invited to were held by churches. The Catholic church is vehemently opposed to the idea of voluntary death.

A prominent Bishop, whom I knew well, told someone, 'If Kochouseph wants to do something like that, why can't he do it in silence by himself? Why does he want to drag a court and a land and the whole people in his way?'

One such forum was organized by the Church in Thrissur. It was a gathering of priests, nuns and activists. In that meeting I made a statement: 'I don't believe we are all happy and healthy just because of God. That is just a reason. Besides that reason, there's human will in the form of technology and medical science that help us survive. My mother had six children; many others at that time had eight or ten kids.

I have only two children because I did a vasectomy. This is the example of human will. This is how humans shape their habitat in order to sustain resources for its own future.'

The audience had a lot of parish opinion leaders who were known and unknown to me. Many were unable to counter my point or justify their fanatic addiction to prolonging human lifetime.

My point was if we can plan our family, why can't we do geriatric planning? There was an uneasy hush in the crowd. I said that this was my wish and the laws of my land should allow me to fulfil it. I wasn't asking anyone to follow my path. The Sub Court rejected my plea. We then moved the High Court. However, after a while I lost interest. In 2011, in Aruna Shanbaug's case, the Supreme Court made a statement that the patient in a condition such as hers (she was on a life support system) can have the liberty to reject medicines and food. That's quite close to an ideal ruling.

Chapter 11

The Big Date

As in any professionally run hospital, Lakeshore too had an Ethics Committee. The spouse of the donor had to appear before the committee to give his or her consent for the donation. This was mandatory. The hospital management also documented the testimony to avoid future confusion or refusal of permissions.

Sheela sat before Dr Aby Abraham and a few other heads of departments. The committee asked her, 'Have you given consent for this?'

Sheela said, 'Even if I don't agree, he will do this. So it's better to agree.'

They realized that she was expressing her true feelings. They wisely advised her to be cautious with such replies when she appeared before the state's official medical committee. She had to have a strong mind by then and give her firm consent.

The hospital management decided that the surgery would take place on the 23 February 2011.

Yet another hurdle remained on my way. I had to obtain official permission from governmental authorities and the Police Commissioner of the city I lived in had to sign my papers. A medical team of experts constituted by the state government was to cross-examine my family and me to understand and assess that the motivation behind the donation was not prejudiced or illegal. As my city fell under the central Kerala domain, the committee sat in the Medical College at Kottayam. There were such committees in Calicut and Thiruvananthapuram as well. This was a mandatory step before a donation of any organ could be made to prevent malpractice.

The chairperson of the committee was the principal of the Medical College. If my memory serves well, there were seven members in the committee. Most of them were senior heads of departments of the college. I was required to explain why I was making the donation and I also had to answer their questions. Sheela and Mithun had to answer and convince the committee that everything was done with the consent of everyone involved. Fr Chiramel had given me enough warnings about this session. He had once failed to win their approval and his wish to donate was rejected.

Fr Chiramel's wish to donate his kidney voluntarily was severely opposed by his church leaders. In the case of a priest, the Bishop had to give the consent, but the Bishop in this case was adamantly opposed to the idea. Fr Chiramel had to convince him first. Understandably, his brother and sister also were opposed to the idea. He somehow managed to convince them as well. However on the day of the meeting of the committee, his brother confessed that Fr Chiramel was so adamant about his wish that he had forced them emotionally to agree to the donation. The medical committee unanimously rejected Fr Chiramel's plea. The priest had to go through the process all over again before the committee gave its final approval.

I took this case as a warning. I had to convince Sheela who was to appear before the committee so before we left for the session I reminded her repeatedly that if the meeting went wrong, my plan would fall flat. I would lose my honour. I told her that if at all she had any difference of opinion, she should keep it aside when giving her answer. She nodded. I could sense her trepidation and I understood her worries. This was a delicate issue and I could not have pressed her much at that stage.

How could I have asked her to keep aside her emotions which were the result of the love between us?

Neither could I have given in to her fears myself. It was a tight-rope walk.

Since the press meet had been held in the previous week, the medical committee members were familiar with my name and wish. A senior lady physician headed the committee.

The session was held at one end of a long hall and the rest of the family had to sit far away. This meant that while they were questioning Sheela, I had no chance to even hear what she was being asked, let alone 'influence' my wife with my presence.

On our appointed day, the committee had to assess thirty to forty cases, recipients or donors coming from remote villages amongst others. I was surprised at the number. When my turn came, we went and sat before the committee. The members had some kind words for me. It was a long table with six or seven people sitting around. Four of us were present, Sheela, Mithun, Jolly and I. A lady was seen taking notes as I answered. They asked me why I was making this donation. They then proceeded to ask if I knew of all the medical and ethical consequences of my action. I answered in the affirmative. They further asked if my family was convinced and were in agreement with my decision. I said they were. They didn't harass me with any more questions. As they knew of the affair through the media, this procedure appeared more like a formality. It took us less than three minutes. However, I knew the committee had rejected several applications before mine. We had to return to the far end of the hall and wait. Then they called Sheela. Her face went pale. She stood up and walked towards the committee members. At the other end of the hall, I sat tense about what she would say. I couldn't hear what they were talking about. Soon after, it was Mithun's turn and then Jolly's.

On our way back, Sheela sat by my side on the back seat of the car while Mithun drove. I looked at Sheela. She looked out of the window watching the city go by. I asked her what they had asked her. She did not utter a word. I smiled. I could understand. To end the awkward silence, Mithun said that they asked him if he had agreed to and understood the possible consequences of my actions. He had said 'yes'. I looked at Sheela again. She still sat with her eyes turned away from me.

Chapter 12

Getting Closer

As the date of my surgery approached, my friends started enquiring if I was growing tense. It was natural to think so. The decision of the committee could come any moment and it could either make it a wonderful day or one where disappointment awaited me.

It was perhaps natural to feel tensed about it, but such worries were not in my nature. Once I had decided on something after much deliberation, I stuck to it, whether I was right or wrong, whether I won or lost. The date, the magic date of 23 February, was to mark my victory in a long-drawn-out battle. It also meant that I would complete a task and carry the burden that lay on my shoulders. The feelings were similar to what I had felt on the day I inaugurated Veegaland after two years of conceptualizing and building it. To me, mathematics comes second to my love for a project. Of course, I would not push for a project that lacks any economic sense. Neither do I cow down before numbers and projections. On the day of the inauguration of Veegaland, I had felt truly vindicated. A vision had passed many tests and was finally ready to be offered to the world. The date of my surgery also presented similar emotions.

Some of the doctors too seemed worried that my anxiety level would possibly go up. On the contrary, I was thrilled. I think this is how we should do our karma. If we find joy in the very act of doing it, then every reward it earns will be that much sweeter. Perhaps due to their kindness, or as a part of their standard practice, my doctors informed me that even though the idea of the surgery had progressed so far, I had every right to reverse my decision and pull out of the donation. I replied I'd rather kill myself than change my word on this. I used the same ploy to silence Sheela. I told her if she made a fuss now over the issue, I would have to commit suicide because the entire state now knew about my intention. In a way I'm grateful to all who stood by me. It showed me the positive outcome of my acts. Some acts can lead others to search within themselves to produce their best attitudes. Love and compassion always spark similar feelings in others. They light lamps of hope in our hearts. This keeps this universe going.

Some friends were not beyond cracking jokes about the matter. One went this way: 'When he dies and goes to heaven,

Pathros [St Peter] will halt Kochouseph saying his body is incomplete with a kidney not yet dead and still working somewhere in Kerala. And they will make him wait at the gates.'

I had a good laugh at such jokes. I usually take things in an easy-going manner. I don't give too much importance to my life or its details, basic ethics aside. However making too much fuss about how we live our lives is generated by religion. Homocentric religions or those that place humans in the centre of the universe, think only from the perspective of humans and make us believe that we are part of God and made in his image.

Does this mean all other living beings are not part of the cosmic force?

Is it not true that we have the power of thought? Isn't it also true that the same power of thinking gave birth to all our problems as well? How does this one faculty make us greater than other forms of life?

We are, after all, just one among many organisms put on this planet. We believe ourselves to be superior and think we have the right to kill any creature. We also make laws. We pretend to assume titles of business tycoons, kings and bishops. However Jesus or Buddha did not do that. They were men of no pretensions as I've learned from the scriptures and texts.

Human beings are not a special creation of God. Yet there are so many differences that drive us apart from one another, wealth, education and opportunities being chief among them. For me, the simple life in a village still held a charm. We had two acres of land in Parapur, my native village. That was my father's property. There was a small tile factory there. We had demolished it and built an old age home that is run by Catholic nuns. There are lush farms and plenty of cattle while the home gets unpolluted organic fruits and vegetables. Whenever we go there, the villagers gift us bundles of bananas. These little things hold value for me. The glitz of modern living or larger than life philosophies do not interest me. This is why I felt that in its core, Naxalism made sense although I did not attach my sympathies to the means Naxalites adopted. We as a system didn't give them enough space and enough dignity. Now I can preach because I have facilities and comfort. I have the affluence of influence and economic ability. Thus I now have the ability to say we must not steal money. Yet if my business saw a steep decline, and I am without means, I am not sure what I would do. I adopt such views in friendly debates, but have noticed that most people dislike listening to such ideas.

Everyone claims India is very religious. Yet India is also quite high on the list of corrupt nations. It's a sign of greed.

Now how can a nation that claims to be full of religious people also be greedy?

I had an old scooter which I used to deliver my handmade stabilizers to shops. This is how ventures are born. This is the natural way to grow. We grow on our own. Some call it hard work; some believe it is determination. It could be both. To me, it is also human will not to succumb to one's own fears.

It's about deciding what we want in life and standing up to face the breeze and the storms alike. Any decision has to have audacity behind it. If not, it will fail.

Sometimes our near and dear ones discourage us due to their love or concern for us. We need to stand by our intuition; we need to protect it. In turn it will protect us. It might take time. Successes come through failures. We need to try several paths to find out what's ours. Since I happened to implement all my plans successfully, friends and people around me believed in my idea of parting with a vital body organ. The faith of those around us comes from their trust in us and our capacity to undertake something and execute it perfectly. There is this trait of adventure and rebellion in me, which I have had from my childhood. If I come across a concept, and I believe it will not stand the test of reason and intuition, then I'll raise questions against it, however popular or dear that concept is to people around me. I enjoy taking up such challenges.

I have a way of seeing the logic in most situations. My father died when he was eighty-six. For most of his life he was healthy and could manage his affairs all by himself. However he had a nasty fall and for a year till his death he was bedridden. He was hospitalized for some time but then the doctors discharged him saying that he was better off at home than in the hospital. During that time I had to leave for the US. He passed away five days after I left. I couldn't return within twenty-four hours so I convinced my siblings to bury him in my absence. I didn't cry because I knew my father had lived a full life.

Why cry for an hour or two and then forget that man, knowing well that death is certain for every being? Why show all those tears? Why must I be sad for a man who lived a full life? Do we really feel broken inside for a man of eighty-six for having died peacefully? Or do we do it as a custom or for the sake of propriety?

This characteristic of mine helped me to analyze such situations and stop worrying.

One day, I was sitting in Dr Aby Abraham's room. Behind him, on the wall, there hung a painting of a man walking on a tight-rope. It spoke volumes on the art of medical science; the art of bringing a man back from the brink of ill health. It also hinted at the risks involved for doctors and patients. Dr Abraham had given me several warnings along with hearty doses of encouragement.

He told me, 'Every surgery carries its risk. It's always 50 per cent.'

I had taken time to digest that truth. A person who fainted at the sight of blood to turning into an organ donor voluntarily must be an amusing fact. I was hospitalized for the first time in my life for my vasectomy and I was a little afraid to undergo that surgery. It took just two hours. When I went into the operation theatre, I was so very anxious about my surgery Now, it seems like a joke.

Chapter 13

Going in

I had once known a man who had been suffering from hernia for four years. He would not go in for a surgery for the fear of dying. As I had undergone a surgery for hernia two years ago, I told him there was nothing to fear. I tried to put some courage into him. He didn't relent. I wondered how he managed with his pain. He said he would rather carry the pain than go through a surgery. That's how fear can freeze us and hold us a prisoner at times.

I, on the other hand, think that we need to look at fear squarely in its eyes. We can stand up to anything that bogs us down and it'll have to go away. Or we draw all the courage in ourselves.

We need to tell ourselves, 'Let me see what happens when I walk through it all.'

Nothing can beat us if we arm ourselves with this attitude. By the end of the journey, we'll have an unflinching sense of accomplishment.

Seven years ago, I was rushed to a hospital. While sitting in the office, I suddenly lost my ability to talk for about a minute. It was a frightening experience. I tried to talk but no words came out. I pressed the buzzer button and someone came in. From my signs those around me figured out my inability to speak. They rushed me to the hospital. On the way I was even feeling a little amused.

How can a man suddenly lose his ability to talk?

At the hospital they diagnosed my problem and said it was due to a micro blood clot that happens for a second or two. I was admitted in the hospital for four days. I learned this condition was called Transient Ischemic Attack (TIA). Apparently, the body dissolves this micro clot by itself.

Wonders of life!

Now that I was on the verge of a major surgery, I had to maintain calm. Perhaps some curiosity was added to the entire process. I had been planning this donation for a long time. If the recipient got ill at the last minute, the surgery would have to be postponed. That remained my only fear. Fortunately, my fears never came true. I kept checking with the doctors if the patient was all right. Joy was well. He was under constant observation and they kept giving him the necessary vitamins to help him stay healthy. Joy was fortunately quite healthy even after the trauma of an ill-functioning kidney. Compared to Valsa, he was in the pink of health. Even during the height of his trauma, he had travelled long distance in a bus from Pala to Kochi to consult a doctor. Joy was admitted in the hospital a week before the surgery to undergo the necessary remaining tests. In the days preceding the surgery, the doctor and I spoke almost twice a day. Mostly I kept in touch with Dr Aby, the nephrologist and the surgeon, Dr George. The nephrologist's role ends once the donor is ready for the donation. The surgeon and anaesthetist then take over.

Even in the final week before the surgery, my siblings checked with me to see if I had had a change of heart. They had to attend countless calls from their friends and relatives and had to answer them on my behalf. I didn't want anyone to visit me at the hospital, so Sheela's sisters and mine visited us prior to us leaving for the procedure. As always, I cheered them with my usual jest. The week before the surgery, Arun and his family flew down from Bengaluru. I wanted them to leave before the surgery as Aarav would insist on playing with me whenever he saw me, and if he found me bedridden he would go sullen. I didn't want that to happen. Arun came back a few days before the surgery after leaving his family back in Bengaluru. Mithun was living in Kochi itself and he was present on the day of the surgery.

I had been asked to get admitted a day before the surgery. So on 22 February, soon after a simple lunch, Sheela and I were driven to the hospital. We were carrying a suitcase each. We were given an executive room, which was big and spacious.

This was, of course, unnecessary. I wouldn't have minded if the room were as spartan as a monastic cell.

The nurses came and went in a procession. There were lots of things to be done it seemed, right from testing blood pressure to asking me pleasant questions. I played along. A reporter–photographer team from *Malayala Manorama* had taken permission to take a picture of Joy and me. That night Dr Aby said I better take a pill to sleep well. I said there was no need for that, but he insisted.

'You're in unfamiliar surroundings among people who are strangers to you. Sometimes, even without you knowing you may get tense. Also, the nurses will keep coming in to give a drip dose or medicines and your sleep may be disturbed. That's not ideal given what's in store for us tomorrow.'

This was a major surgery. I remember clearly what my anaesthetist told me. He said, 'It is a process.' After the surgery I won't be allowed to walk away just like that. I would be kept in the Intensive Care Unit under observation for a day. I wasn't happy about that. I simply wanted to give away my kidney and be driven home to rest. I wanted a break. Understanding that could not be done, I relented.

When an impending surgery knocks on the door, it is said that patients begin feeling the body balancing hormones produced by the kidneys as they create a feeling of imbalance in the body. Thus a donor must be kept under observation for a day.

After the day of observation, I was given something to

drink. It had an odd taste. The doctors said it acted as a laxative before the surgery. Cleaning the bowels keeps the patient safe so that he or she doesn't need to relieve themselves during the surgery. Some might vomit in the process. If that happens, the vomit enters the lungs and complicates the procedure. Similarly, the sleeping pill was to make sure that the patient has a deep sleep the night before the surgery to ensure that his systems works perfectly during the operation.

In the hospital room, while I sat on the bed Sheela unpacked our things, her face shrivelled with intense worry. What would happen to her beloved husband when the hospital trolley takes him away? This thought was painted on her face. I could sense her depression. She appeared tired. I knew that she had had several sleepless nights fearing for my life. The circles under her eyes were darkening.

Apparently, Sheela was the one who went through all the pressures. She is a loving and sentimental woman. She was quite emotional when younger; perhaps, life with a hard nut like me had shaped and changed her character in some ways. My self-reliance, determination and faith in my willpower must have rubbed off on her as well. Willing or unwilling, she had to stand by her man. She also was the one who would lose the most if something untoward happened to me. I felt overwhelming love for her. The previous night at home, I had seen her saying her prayers with tears in her eyes. I hugged her and told her to stay calm.

'I will come back,' I whispered into her ears.

It was then that her eyes got back some radiance. I could only hope she would draw some more courage from the cosmic sources she trusted.

We had dinner together. Soon after a nurse came in and gave me the sleeping pill. It would start working on me after two hours. A little later, a male nurse came in to shave the hair on my body, a mandatory procedure. Soon after I fell asleep peacefully.

Around five in the morning, a nurse came in to fill the drip bag. I woke up fresh at about 6 a.m. Sheela was already awake. I'm not sure if she had slept at all. At about 7 a.m., I was served some black tea. Soon after someone brought an IV fluid to maintain the energy level of my body. I wasn't supposed to eat anything before the surgery. Finally, they said I would be shifted to the operation theatre by 8 a.m. By then, Mithun, Arun and Joshna came in. It was good to see them because I was worried about Sheela. Now she had some company to share her angst. As for me, I was far from being tense. I was glad the procedure was happening. As the day bloomed, I guess it all began becoming a little hazy. The doctors had mixed a small dose of a sleeping drug in the drip they gave me early in the morning. There were other surgeries scheduled for the day. Mine was the first.

Around 7:45 a.m., a team of nurses arrived in my room. They gave me a green robe to wear. I was to remove every piece of cloth on me including my underwear. Sheela had taken off my rings and chain and my spectacles. Someone brought in a stretcher trolley and I got on it. Sheela and my sons were looking at me intently. I could very well walk, but the attendants and nurses disallowed it. We were on the eighth floor and the operation theatre was a few floors down. I was taken into a lift and then the trolley was wheeled through several corridors. We finally turned into a room and halted before a door with a board that said, 'Operation Theatre'.

This was the last point where my dear ones could accompany me. I saw Sheela was almost in tears. I didn't know what to say. Joshna, Mithun and Arun stood by trying their best to pacify her. I'm not sure if they themselves were steady enough to bid me 'goodbye'. I raised my hand to them. Then someone pushed the trolley inside. The room had several personnel in uniforms, waiting and ready to lift me up onto another stretcher brought in from the theatre. I was quickly taken in, with the door shutting on my wife, sons and daughter-in-law.

I wanted to see the operation theatre properly. As soon as I was taken in, I saw the anaesthetist approaching me and looking down at me as I lay on the stretcher. He placed his warm palms on my forehead and asked me, 'Are you ready?'

I nodded.

His assistants handed over the syringe. He patted me, placed the needle on my right arm, smiled and said 'Sleep well'. Then he pressed it into my flesh.

I faintly heard him telling me, 'Don't worry, we will take care of you.'

I remember the big white lights. I remember eight or nine men and women standing around me dressed in green cloaks. Their faces were covered with surgical masks. I could only see their eyes pouring down at me. It was then that everything started to blur. Everything started to slip away and I began to wonder why I was there, in the operation theatre.

What had brought me to that surgical table under those bright lights?

It had all started with a thought that had floated into my mind about eight months ago. One tiny thought. In the intervening months, it had grown and now I lay naked under a green cloak, surrounded by strangers wearing masks and uniforms. I began slipping, falling into a white phantom land under the blinding light. I wondered how big the knife was going to be. I thought of my beloved wife Sheela.

I mumbled to myself, 'Lie calm, lie calm, everything's going to be fine.'

That was 23 February 2011.

Chapter 14

Back to My Senses

When I became conscious, twenty-two hours had passed. It was about 5:30 p.m. when I woke up. There were a few tubes running in and out of my body. I had no pain due to the painkillers I had been administered. I realized then that the team of surgeons had removed my left kidney and safely transplanted it in Joy. The donation was complete. I was happy that I was still alive, and my wish had materialized. That mattered more to me than anything else. I looked around and saw Sheela overjoyed to see me conscious again. So were Arun and Mithun. We held each other's hands tightly.

They said the doctors had allowed them to see me around 3 p.m. on the day of the surgery, around five hours after the surgery. Sheela and Mithun had seen me nodding my head at them and even answered some of their questions. I do not remember anything. Then I saw Fr Chiramel standing in the corner of the room with a big smile. At the same time, he was also almost in tears. We clasped our palms. Our wish had been granted. Two men with a single kidney each, stood happily holding each other's hands, as if we were on top of the world.

Three days after the surgery, I was discharged. They told me not to undertake any travel right away as the body would be weak after the surgery. On the seventh day I was told to come back to the hospital to remove the dressing on the wound. During my visit, I was told that the cut made during the surgery had healed and the dressing was removed.

When one goes through such a major surgery, the entire body is sedated with strong anaesthesia. Even the lungs are sedated. During the surgery it would have worked artificially. Wounds heal in three days but lungs that have been operated artificially for four to five hours of surgery tend to become lethargic as their muscles have stopped operating during the said duration.

Thus they gave me a lung power refreshing blower with three balls. I was told to blow inside it at home, till the tiny balls in the blower rose—an exercise to bring back the strength in my lungs.

On the eighth day after the surgery, I went to office. The staff were surprised by my speedy recovery. We held a meeting in the hall. Almost all the employees gathered there. When I narrated how it all went, one of them fainted. There were a lot of questions. These pertained to the surgery—if I was experiencing pain, if I had felt discomfort during the surgery, what was I eating, could I have an occasional brandy, and more. I answered all of them patiently. I sat feeling happy that my strange wish had bloomed for the good of all.

A few days after the surgery, I got a call from a friend. His voice was shaky. He said that he had come to know that a public interest group in Kerala was planning to move the court against me. I asked him what my crime was. He was unsure how to put the news across to me. I encouraged him because I was more amused than surprised. He said the group believed that my surgery was a media hype I had created. It was believed I had not undergone any surgery and I still had both my kidneys with me. Now I wanted to know more. My friend said the group was going to ask the court to constitute a medical committee to examine me thoroughly and check if I had really donated the kidney. I had a hearty laugh on hearing this. That must have put my friend at ease. I said that would be wonderful since I would then be in the papers once again and that would give us more opportunities to spread the message that donation of vital organs was important and the need of the hour. Fr Chiramel too called me when he heard about this group's move, raging over the phone against the group. I had to pacify him after some effort.

Anyone in our shoes would have felt injured at such a response. We had no intentions to manipulate anyone. We only believed in doing things our way, for a good cause. I still believe in old-fashioned values of straightforwardness, integrity and honesty. I trust people and believe in the best they have to offer. Harsh responses like these from some people did not hamper my positive nature. My sense of hope in human beings is too strong and can bear all the suspicion that came by way.

Later, having nothing to do because I had to undergo rest for two weeks, I sat in my living room thinking about people around me. I believe people are good at heart and bitter experiences in life make them think in extreme ways. It's true that there is a lot of hype around us in the media. Leaders in politics, trade and show business do sometimes resort to hype. There are people who generate an unreasonable amount of publicity. People might have been already miffed by it. Some could have counted me with such people. I ended up justifying them rather than condemning their actions. Later, when some reporters came over, I deliberately pulled up my T-shirt to show the surgery cut in my belly. That, I hoped, would put all speculation to rest.

Sometimes people react to things a little too enthusiastically. Journalist generally exaggerates somebody's positive trait. It's the other way when it comes to slandering. If somebody makes an error, the media scrutinizes it immensely. By donating a kidney I never imagined getting such a massive response from society. People began to look at me as somebody who breaks conventions. Wherever I went, they stared at me; I was used to be looked upon as a familiar face. Now, I began seeing incredulous looks blending with a sense of admiration. I had not wished for all this.

Three weeks later at the passport office, a man came and touched my feet. A similar incident took place at a meeting at the Rotary Club where I had been invited to attend a large conference. Someone came and kissed my palms. While uncomfortable with such gestures, I would have felt gratified if people would have offered to become donors, giving meaning to my act.

Soon after, I began getting a lot of calls. Several invitations came my way to attend meetings to honour and interact with me. I attended a couple of them. Soon it started to bother me as I had to travel far and wide. However, soon I found a grand opportunity in this. It occurred to me that I could charge a fee for such talks. It wasn't for myself but to fund charitable causes. The second advantage was that I benefitted from forums where I could explain and spread the right information about kidney donation. The questions asked in these forums worried me. These ranged from the basic to the disbelieving.

Are donors required to take medicines for the rest of their lives?

No. I had to reassure them. The only medicines which I had to take were antibiotics for the first five days after the surgery and some vitamin tablets for the next ten.

Other questions were like whether I could eat pork or continue drinking alcohol. I ate all that as modestly even before my donation. I have always been an occasional drinker.

Three months after the surgery when I visited the hospital for a mandatory check-up, I received a lot of love from the doctors and nurses. They tested my blood and urine samples, told me that my case has been happily concluded and that I shouldn't be seen anywhere near the hospital again. We had a good laugh that day. The doctors told me to forget that I ever had undergone a surgery and that I could go on living as I had earlier. I happily took the advice and went home.

Chapter 15

The Butterfly Effect

My doctor observed that my donation had a ripple effect on society. They were used to seeing a lot of hesitancy on the part of kith and kin when it came to the question of donating a kidney to their ailing relative, be it to a husband, wife, brother, sister, son or daughter. Thanks to the wide and positive media coverage people had begun to shed their fears. The thought that a successful man who donated his kidney continues to be successful and healthy motivated them to tread on my path. If that ripple grows far and wide, serving the ailing and deserving ones, I guess I would be a happier person.

This is one area where even the most determined ones give up after a while. Willing persons do come in to donate, but in a few days after their close relatives or even life partners interfere, the potential donor vanishes. Most often, they are discouraged with unnecessary fears. That's one major stumbling block for potential donors. A lot of awareness still needs to spread. A lot of questions still bother us.

Why shouldn't someone be free to donate his organs? Why shouldn't there be a paid donor system approved by the authorities? Why make it all a Herculean task to get a donated organ?

These are not simple questions.

There are larger issues of values, ethics and possibilities of exploitation involved. In a poor country like India, the possibility of donors exploiting the ailing and desperate could create a chaotic environment. A State can't obviously deal with accusations of participating in marketing of human body parts. There is an important question of human dignity involved here. At the same time, a form of an open window system should be followed to save a large number of waiting recipients who already have donor agreements in place.

About six months after my surgery, I read a story in a newspaper that gladdened me immensely.

A twenty-nine-year-old man named Joshy in Wayanad donated his kidney to a woman in his town. He was a signboard painter and a local party worker. He hadn't called me or Fr Chiramel. He never offered to talk or ask questions as many of us do. He just went ahead and donated his organ. We traced him and spoke to him and was very impressed. He was a daily wage worker and he had silently performed

114 • *The Gift*

a noble deed without grand announcements though he had heard about our donations.

I told him, 'Young man, I did it when I turned sixty, you're hardly thirty, which is extraordinary.'

He had a new-born daughter and his wife had supported him wholeheartedly. He just smiled as he replied. His easy attitude about the whole affair was quite disarming. Joshy had come to know of a poor woman in his town in need of a kidney and just gave his organ to her. Joshy had always been inclined to perform some social service and as a party worker he did reach out to people. However his concern for others was beyond petty political leanings. He was a true Samaritan who worried more about his neighbour's problems than his own. We gifted him two lakh rupees from the Kidney Federation Fund to show our solidarity with his act of great compassion.

For Fr Chiramel, it was time to look into the chain donation he had arranged. Jolly had promised to give hers to another man. His wife had agreed to donate to yet another man. A magnificent chain was already in place, a chain of promise to help each other to live and let live. Nothing was easy about this. Even my decision had come after a prolonged contemplation and dedication of several weeks and months to see myself through it. Similarly, Fr Chiramel spent days and nights to find the most needy recipient and then convince the donor to donate so that the chain got going. At each point, willingness had to be created and lack of awareness had to be combated. This was a time-consuming effort.

Nothing is easy about human decisions; particularly when it comes to opening one's body for others. After several months, a chain had been formed. The man who was to get Jolly's kidney had been on dialysis. Patients on dialysis turn weak as their kidney functions in an improper way. Since they are highly medicated, their blood vessels became thin. Such patients are highly fragile. Sadly, the man who was to receive Jolly's kidney passed away before the transplant could be done.

A shocking majority of kidney patients die of non-availability of kidneys. However, in this case, this man had been found by Fr Chiramel and was offered a kidney. He was offered life. He must have gone through days and nights of pain and trouble with the hope that finally he had been chosen to be given a new life. However the ways of our bureaucracy are strange. Officers take a terribly long time to move papers and there are a lot of bureaucratic hassles. Concerns are understandable, but legalities have turned into stumbling blocks. Officers seem to believe a lot more in red tape than a breathing man. It's only cases for them—a man dead and gone is one file less to be processed. That's how government machinery works.

There are kind people everywhere and not everyone is apathetic but everyone thinks of the system first and the spirit of the law later. No one wants to take bruises in the name of altruism. No one even considers the need of the other in any earnestness. That has become the way of the world.

It was a great setback to us. The man died when a chance to get life was within reach. With his death Fr Chiramel's chain was broken. In a few weeks, another patient in the chain died.

Still, the human spirit surprises us with its inherent goodness. In this case, though the man who was to receive the kidney died, his wife did not go back on her word. Fr Chiramel, who had taken the news of the man's death with such agony, set out to fix a new chain and to get it going. Now four donors were ready in the first chain as well as four recipients. More were slowly being added in a second chain.

At the end of the day, what did I learn out of all this?

I learned a lesson. That an action is a hundred times more effective than preaching. However much money or time or words or energy I or anyone had spent to popularize the idea of organ donation, it wouldn't have made such an impact. When somebody stepped in to lie on a surgery table, the wave of response became immense. This is what they call the 'butterfly effect'. It is attributed to a meteorologist named Edward Norton Lorenz. It suggests that the flapping of a butterfly's wings in South America could affect the weather in Texas.

I love this idea. It simply means that even a tiny action in one part of the world can have a bigger effect on another part. I hope our actions for the good of all have a butterfly effect on the world, so that it becomes a better place to live in.

Months after the surgery, a child walked up to me and

asked, 'Sir, if there's anything you have gained from your organ donation, can you tell me what that is?'

I was a little surprised at this unique query from a girl. I've faced a lot of questions, but mostly from adults. Here was this child standing in front of me and wanting to know what I had gained out of all this. Perhaps she was prompted by her parents who stood a little away, beaming proudly. I took a moment to think of how to put it to her in the way she would understand.

Then I said, 'My dear, when I gave away a kidney, I got immensely richer in my heart.'

She understood and smiled shyly. Then we shook hands and went our different ways. A moment later, I turned around to see the little girl holding her parents' hands and skipping away merrily—like a butterfly that could change tomorrow's world.

Annexure

Organ Donation in India: Legal Regulations and Restrictions

In India, the removal, storage and transplantation of human organs for therapeutic purposes are regulated by the Transplantation of Human Organs Act, 1994 and the Rules thereunder, namely the Transplantation of Human Organs Rules, 1995. The primary object of the Act is to prevent commercial dealings in human organs and regulate matters connected therewith or incidental thereto.

The Act restricts the removal of a human organ from the body of a donor, before his death, and transplantation into the body of a recipient unless the donor is a 'near relative' of the recipient. A 'near relative' for the purposes of the law include a spouse, son, daughter, father, mother, brother or sister. If any donor authorizes the removal of his human organs before his death for transplantation into the body of a recipient, not being a near relative, by reason of affection or attachment towards the recipient or for any other special reasons, the law stipulates that such human organ shall not be removed and transplanted without the prior approval of a duly constituted authorization committee, comprising of members nominated by the government. The donor and the recipient are to make a joint application and the authorization committee has to hold an inquiry and satisfy itself that the applicants have complied with all legal regulations and requirements before an approval is given.

When the proposed donor and recipient are not near relatives, the authorization committee has to evaluate the following:

a) That there is no commercial transaction between the donor and recipient, specifically taking into consideration an explanation as to the link between them and the circumstances which lead to the donation and the reasons as to why the donor wishes to donate.

b) That there is no middle man or tout involved.

c) The financial status of both the donor and the recipient with appropriate evidence of their vocation and income for the previous three financial years, to evaluate if there is any gross disparity between the two, leading to a commercial transaction.

d) That the donor is not a drug addict or a known person with criminal record.

e) That the next of kin of the proposed donor is interviewed and any strong views or disagreements or objection of such kin recorded and taken note of.

Though the object of the legal regulations is laudable, it is generally felt that it has placed considerable obstacles in the process of organ donation, particularly for the common man. For the sake of evaluation of the above circumstances, to prevent commercial dealings, considerable documents and proof are insisted upon by the authorization committees before granting approval, even in emergent cases. Further, the process itself is time-consuming and given the considerable time spent in procuring all necessary certificates and documents from various government authorities, the very object of organ donation—to save a life, is defeated.

www.ingramcontent.com/pod-product-compliance
Lightning Source LLC
Chambersburg PA
CBHW031945190326
41519CB00007B/670

* 9 7 8 8 1 2 9 1 3 9 5 9 7 *